THE MAKING OF A PICKY EATER

How We're Creating a Nation of Picky Eaters
and What You Can Do About It

Beth Robeson
Charlene Ross
illustrations by Lisa Boys

Dedication:

To Brad Robeson for tolerating years of me sneaking away
to write while everyone else was at the beach during our
family vacations.

Strategic3 Publishing

ISBN 978-0-9863603-0-5

Table of Contents

Foreword

Raising kids is hard work, really hard, so cut yourself some slack, and don't get discouraged. Trying to raise healthy kids in a world where junk food is lurking around every corner is often an overwhelming task. It will feel like it's not working some of the time—you'll have both breakthroughs and setbacks. My very picky eater is now 17 and he doesn't even think of himself as a picky eater. Even more importantly, he limits the amount of sugar he consumes, all on his own!

I remember on numerous occasions throughout my son's childhood years, wanting to take them out for ice cream as a special treat. But they'd usually been given so much sugar, cakes, cookies, candy, day glow drinks etc., throughout the day that I feared adding to that crazy mix with a family outing to the ice cream store.

The goal is to support your child when they're home and you have more control over what's presented to them. Then, when they're away from home, run interference for them, to the best of your ability without making yourself crazy.

We had a wonderful literature teacher at the kids' home school program, who kept several big jars of candy in her classroom. My child, who shared my sweet tooth, was coming home from school every day with Skittles and Jolly Ranchers stuffed in his pockets.

I spoke with his teacher about it and the director of the program. They told me that my son was going to be exposed to candy his whole life and he needed to learn to control his sweet tooth. This is something I have personally spent years trying to do for myself and have always failed miserably. If it's sweet and sitting there staring at me, I'm going to eat it, probably sooner rather than later!

I shared with them over time, that by having the candy in the room every day they were in fact teaching kids about diet and nutrition. They were teaching them that candy should be a normal part of your day. I shared that childhood diabetes rates have tripled since the 70's and that what kids eat when they are young has a profound effect on what they eat as an adult. I mentioned that there are lots of other beautiful and healthy ways to spoil or reward kids that are just as fun.

The next school year, a wonderful thing happened. The teacher had removed the candy and instead had set up a beautiful tea station in her room! She had an eclectic selection of mugs and a wide variety of teas to choose from and the kids' could enjoy the aroma and warmth of a hot cup of tea while they learned about the enchanting world of literature.

When my oldest son graduated, the teacher came up to me on graduation day and said, "I just want to tell you,

you were right about the candy and I want to thank you for bringing it to my attention." What a wonderful compliment from an amazing teacher, one who gave both my boys a deep love for a wide variety of literature. It just goes to show you, we each have our gifts and talents and we can all learn from each other.

—Beth Robeson

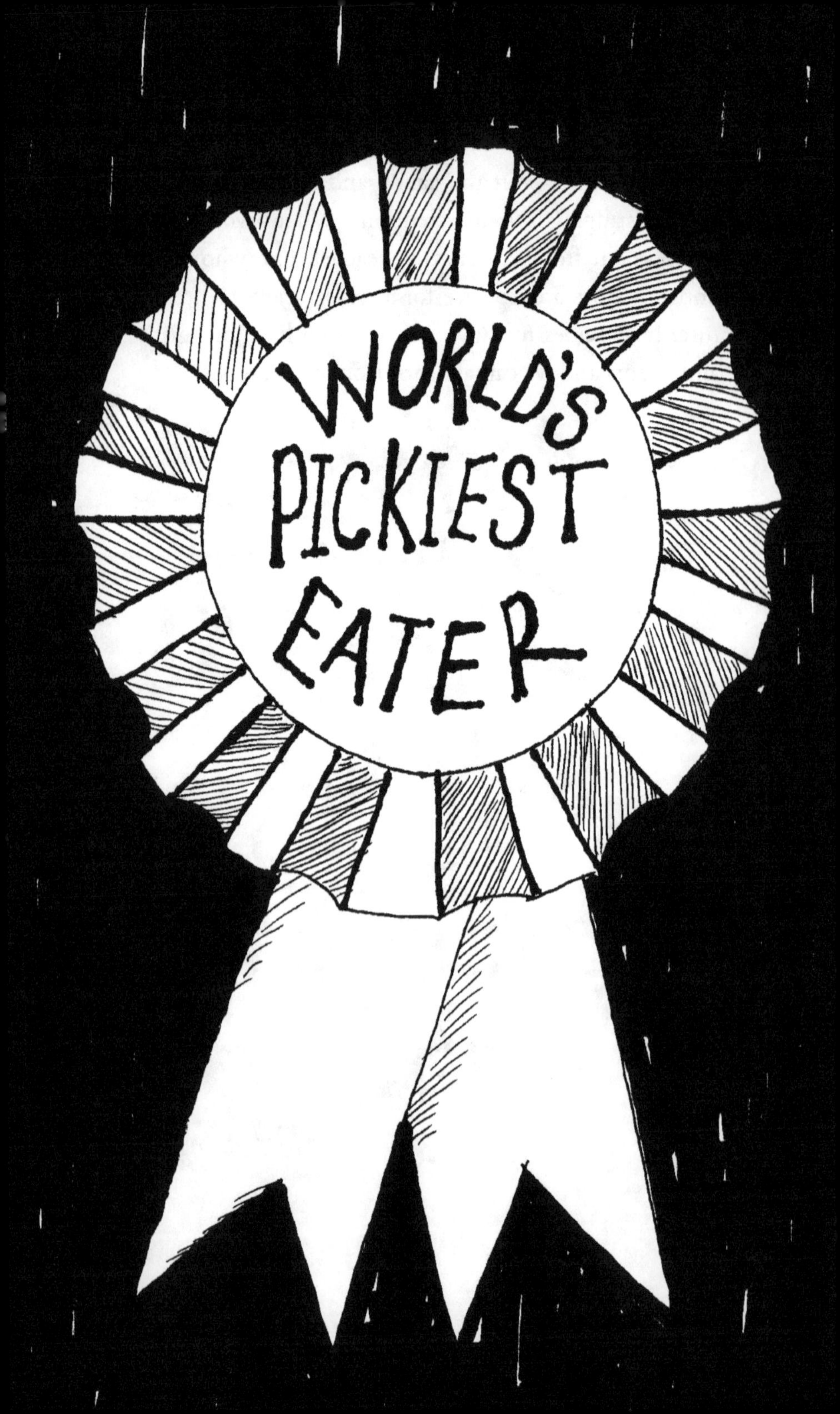
WORLD'S
PICKIEST
EATER

Prove It: How Picky Eaters Are Made Not Born

Parents all over the country are unknowingly creating generations of picky eaters.

That's a controversial statement, but one I'm betting you'll agree with once you've finished this book. Don't worry: as the pages unfold, you'll find no guilt trips, no stress, no blaming anyone or dreary projections. This book is about enjoying life more, enjoying your kids more, and enjoying food more! So before you roll your eyes at me (or after, if you already have), grab your reading glasses and let's get started.

Kids are Born With Sensitive Taste Buds.

Yes, some kids are born with sensitive taste buds, which means they may be hesitant to try new foods and it may take them longer to try and/or warm up to new foods. However, it's what you do with them over the next eighteen years that will determine whether you wind up with a picky eater, a gourmet chef, or something in between.

The "Experts" Need to Rethink Their Numbers!

It takes way longer than most parents realize to get kids with sensitive taste buds to become comfortable with a new food. It certainly takes longer than the experts suggest. Most parents give up after the first two or three tries, while "experts" will tell you it takes as many as fifteen tries of a new food before a child will develop a taste for it.

Fifteen tries?!

For a picky eater that number is way off! Fifteen tries is for quitters!

It took me three years to get my son to eat a salad even after I put a small one in front of him several nights a week for the whole three years. If I were to lowball it, I'd say it took me 468 tries to get him to eat that darn salad! Fifteen tries – Pffft!

Do you have that kind of stamina? Sure you do! Don't make extra work for yourself. It was only a bite or two that I put on his plate, but by doing so he learned salads were just part of dinner. One day sitting in my father's motor home I put a salad in front of him just like everybody else and BAM He just started eating it. I didn't say a word.

It took me sixteen years to get my son to eat papaya. He likes other fruits. Why didn't I just give up after say five or ten years? Because papaya is probably the most nutritious fruit on the planet. Learning to like it put another awesome weapon in his arsenal of disease fighting tools. Now he'll be eating papaya for the rest of his life.

Just remember - your secret weapon is persistence. (Coupled with a large glass of wine.)

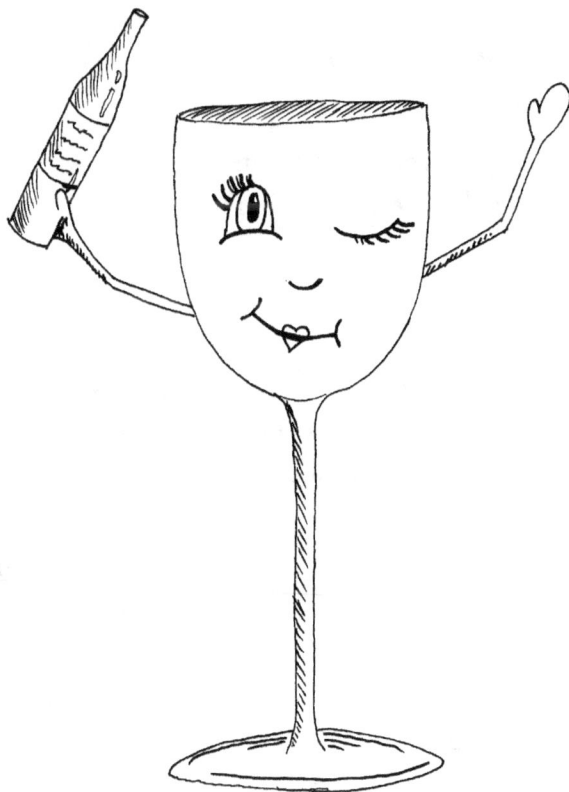

The Dinnertime Battle Ground

Parents of picky eaters try really hard to get their children to eat their vegetables: they cajole, threaten, bribe, and even trick their kids into trying new foods. The problem is, this creates an adversarial relationship between you and your child, between your child and vegetables (or whatever else you are trying to get them to eat), and between your child and dinnertime.

This is the opposite of what you want to achieve. I mean, who wants to sit down to an unpleasant food battle every night? It's enough to make you want to give up on dinner time, throw some chicken nuggets in the microwave, skip the wine and head straight for the freezer vodka instead.

If you want your child to develop a lifetime of healthy eating habits they need to see healthy foods and mealtime as an enjoyable experience, and so do you!

The "Mini-Me" Syndrome!

Some parents of picky eaters were picky eaters themselves, so they sympathize with their "mini-me's" and carry on a generation of picky eater traditions. Don't let your expectations around meals, vegetables, or treats impact what you teach your child about food. You'll be amazed at how different their perspective will be if you offer them frozen peas as a treat when they are little, or blanched broccoli and ranch dressing as a snack, or steamed vegetables for breakfast. Sure steamed vegetables for breakfast sounds weird, but they have no way of knowing that it's weird unless you tell them. You might even surprise yourself and find you enjoy it too!

I Saw it With My Own Eyes!

I've been working with picky eaters for 20 years and I've watched picky eaters fall in love with new healthy foods over and over again, often to the complete surprise and shock of their parents. I've learned that by giving them the chance, the independence, and the right type of en-couragement, they'll discover lots of wonderful things they just love to eat.

The trick is to fall back, regroup, and try a whole new approach to eating healthy - a positive one that focus-es on satisfaction and enjoyment, not deprivation and dinnertime battles. That's what this book is about. Kids are smart, smart enough to understand that it matters what they put into their bodies. It can't be a battle or a power struggle; they have to own it for themselves. And this book will show you how to help them do just that!

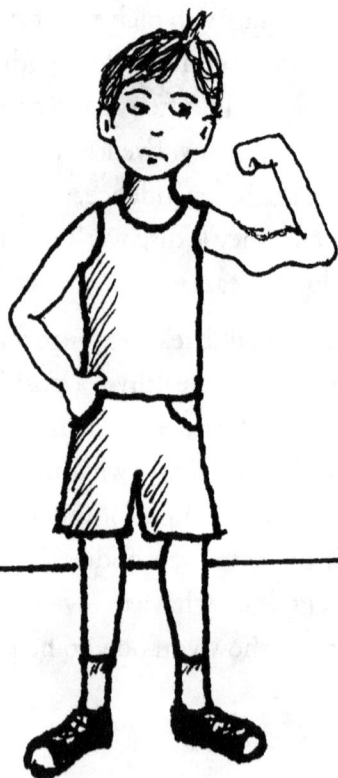

The Problem with Picky

Is it really a problem that we have a society full of picky eaters? After all, mac & cheese and chicken nuggets are easy to prepare and the only thing these kids will eat, so what's the big deal? In the next few pages, I'm going to suggest that it IS a problem, and here's why...

Picky Eaters on Steroids!

Historically, if a child was a picky eater, they were only picky about a small number of foods like beets, brussels sprouts or fish. They ate lots of other healthy whole foods, because when Mom made dinner that was all there was to eat. Making dinner was a time consuming process so Mom didn't have the option of just popping up and making you some chicken nuggets or ordering you whatever you wanted at the fast food restaurant if you didn't like the pot roast.

There were no kids' meals. There was just dinner, and you ate it. Everyone ate it. Now, because of the convenience of fast and processed foods, parents are making their kids whatever they want to avoid confrontation at dinner. As a result, picky eaters are eating the same things over and over and over. This means that instead of being picky about 2-3 foods, they only *eat* 2-3 foods! And, unfortunately, these foods are usually processed and not really food at all. (Have you ever actually seen what's inside of a chicken nugget? The list of 25 ingredients is bigger than the nugget! I make homemade chicken nuggets with one ingredient—you guessed it—chicken.

This brings us to our next important point...

No Real Food!

Processed foods, while delicious, aren't really foods. They're just designed to look and taste like food. For the most part, the nutrients, fiber, vitamins, minerals, antioxidants, enzymes, phytochemicals and anything that was good for you have been processed out of them.

It doesn't mean you can't eat processed foods once in a while, we all have our vices, but it's not a good idea to try living off them, which a lot of picky eaters do.

Processed foods also come in all shapes and sizes and are often touted by the food industry as the healthiest items in the grocery store.

Take your typical "whole grain" bread for example. It might start with a little whole grain, but it's basically as nutritionally void as white flour when they are done with it.

To make matters worse, caramel color is added to make it look brown, as well as wood pulp, a substitution for the fiber they've removed. This allows them to list fiber on the package. Wood pulp, shockingly, does not work the same in the body as fiber from food. The it is topped off with lots of other non-food ingredients like dough conditioners, preservatives, flavorings, and the now infamously added sugar. You might not recognize it as sugar in the ingredients list because the processed food manufactures have developed 56 different names for sugar to throw you off, but if it's a processed food, chances are they've added sugar, since 80% of processed foods now contain added sugar. Real whole grain bread has four ingredients: stone ground whole-wheat flour, water, salt, and yeast. That's it.

Start taking a look at the ingredients list on the bread you buy and on other processed foods. If it has more than three or four ingredients, put it back on the shelf. You can sometimes find a high quality bread in the freezer section or at a local baker who makes real bread. For a great example of a true bread baker check out Blue Oven Bakery at blueovenbakery.com, they are true bread bakers. Look for the term "Stone-ground whole-wheat flour" in the ingredients list.

Here's a shocker… Personally, I would rather give my child a loaf of white bread from a local baker than a loaf of "wheat" bread loaded with unknown artificial ingredients and added sugar.

BEWARE: The food manufacturers are doing everything in their power to throw you off the path of real food. Here are just a few examples:

Wheat Flour: Once parents started looking for whole wheat flour, the processed food manufactures started calling white flour, "wheat flour," White flour technically comes from wheat, so they can get away with it, but it doesn't change the fact that it's just plain old white flour that they started calling "wheat flour."

Stone ground whole wheat flour is what you really want. More expensive? Yes. Less convenient? Yep. Totally worth it? You betcha!

Fruit Sweetened: When the dangers of sugar were becoming well known, parents started looking for fruit sweetened products. So what did the food manufactures do? Create a line of products sweetened with real fruit? Nope. They created an expensive form of sugar water that the FDA let them call "fruit juice sweetened." They've made and continue to make boatloads of money off of "fruit juice sweetened" products. But it's just sugar.

Building a Flimsy Foundation

Since picky eaters don't eat a diverse or densely nutritious diet they are more susceptible to colds, asthma, and other more serious diseases like cancer and diabetes. As your child eats and grows over the years, they will use the nutrients in real food to build strong muscles, brain tissue, bones, and an effective immune system. If they are living off a diet of processed foods, where are they getting these building blocks? It's just like the story of the three little pigs. The materials you use determine the strength of your house.

Where will they get the highest quality building blocks? From these 6 things:

- Lots of vegetables
- Meats (not processed meats)
- Fish
- Fruits and Berries
- Nuts and Seeds
- Real whole grains like brown rice and whole oats.

Home Cooking Gets the Shaft

Because picky eaters won't eat what's made for dinner, making dinner becomes an unpleasant experience. Who wants to put hours of work into cooking a meal and then have your child offer up a big, "yuck?" What a miserable experience. How far would Michelangelo have gotten on the Sistine Chapel if the priest offered up "yuck" after every few strokes of the brush? The good news is that you can actually teach your child to appreciate the food you make and banish "yuck" from your life, instead receiving a big, "Thanks Mom!" Now you're cooking!

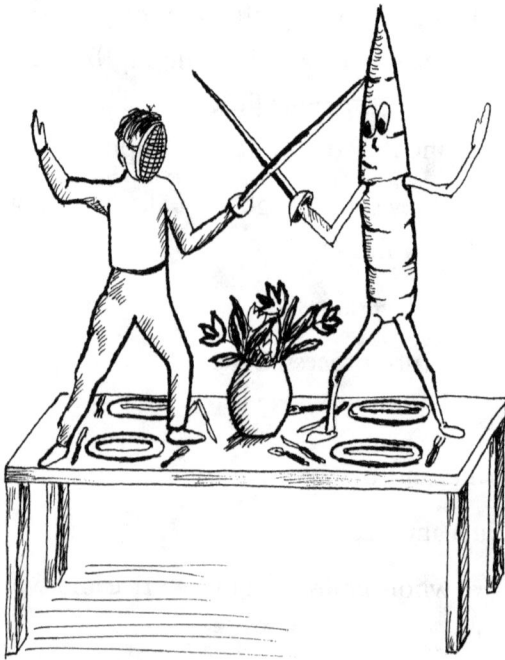

Mealtime Battles

Another problem created by picky eating is the fact that it creates mealtime battles and power plays that make dinner time an unpleasant experience instead of an enjoyable time with family. If mealtime becomes stressful for both the parents and the kids, filled with battles over how many bites of broccoli Junior has to choke down, the precious little time we have with our kids is wasted. Mealtime can and should be a pleasant experience.

Fear of Family & Friend Get Togethers

Sadly, picky eaters are often stressed about eating at family gatherings, having dinner at a friend's house, or trying a new restaurant with Grandma and Grandpa. Who needs that? Eating with friends or trying new things should be fun, and it can be, if you do a few simple things to train their sensitive taste buds to appreciate new foods.

Long Term Health Issues

Lastly, and the biggest concern if you have a picky eater, is that what you eat as a child impacts your diet for the rest of your life. It's much harder to change your eating habits as an adult than as a child, and a poor diet means a greater likelihood of long-term health issues such as high cholesterol, high blood pressure, digestive issues, and cancer. Processed foods loaded with hidden sugar and void of nutrients are a double whammy, because while the sugar damages your body and causes disease, the lack of nutrients gives you nothing to fight back with.

Processed foods are loaded with hidden sugar. (That's why they taste so good!) Sugar causes inflammation in the body. Inflammation has now been linked with all the major diseases we currently struggle with in westernized societies: cancer, heart disease, diabetes, and even Alzheimer's disease.

There are numerous factors that affect the rates of cancer and other diseases, but there is no question that diet plays a major role. The good news is that whole foods like sweet potatoes, broccoli, and green leafy vegetables have built-in disease fighting tools that your body uses to keep you healthy; that's why it's so important.

Summary:

What your child eats is the foundation of their health. It impacts everything from their brain development to their bone strength and their anxiety level. That's why picky eating is dangerous. One of the greatest gifts you can give your child is the gift of health, and if you think feeding your child a healthy diet in today's environment is a challenge, you're right. However, it's nothing in comparison to the challenge of a child or family member faced with a dangerous illness.

The key is to take it slowly.

If you're going to get your kids to eat healthfully, it has to be fun and they have to own it. That's the only way you get there. It can't be stressful or combative, and it can't be a lot of hard work or you'll both give up. The next step is to take a whole new approach to eating healthy, one that's rewarding and fun for both you and your child. Before we do though, let's take a humorous look at how you'd go about creating a picky eater.

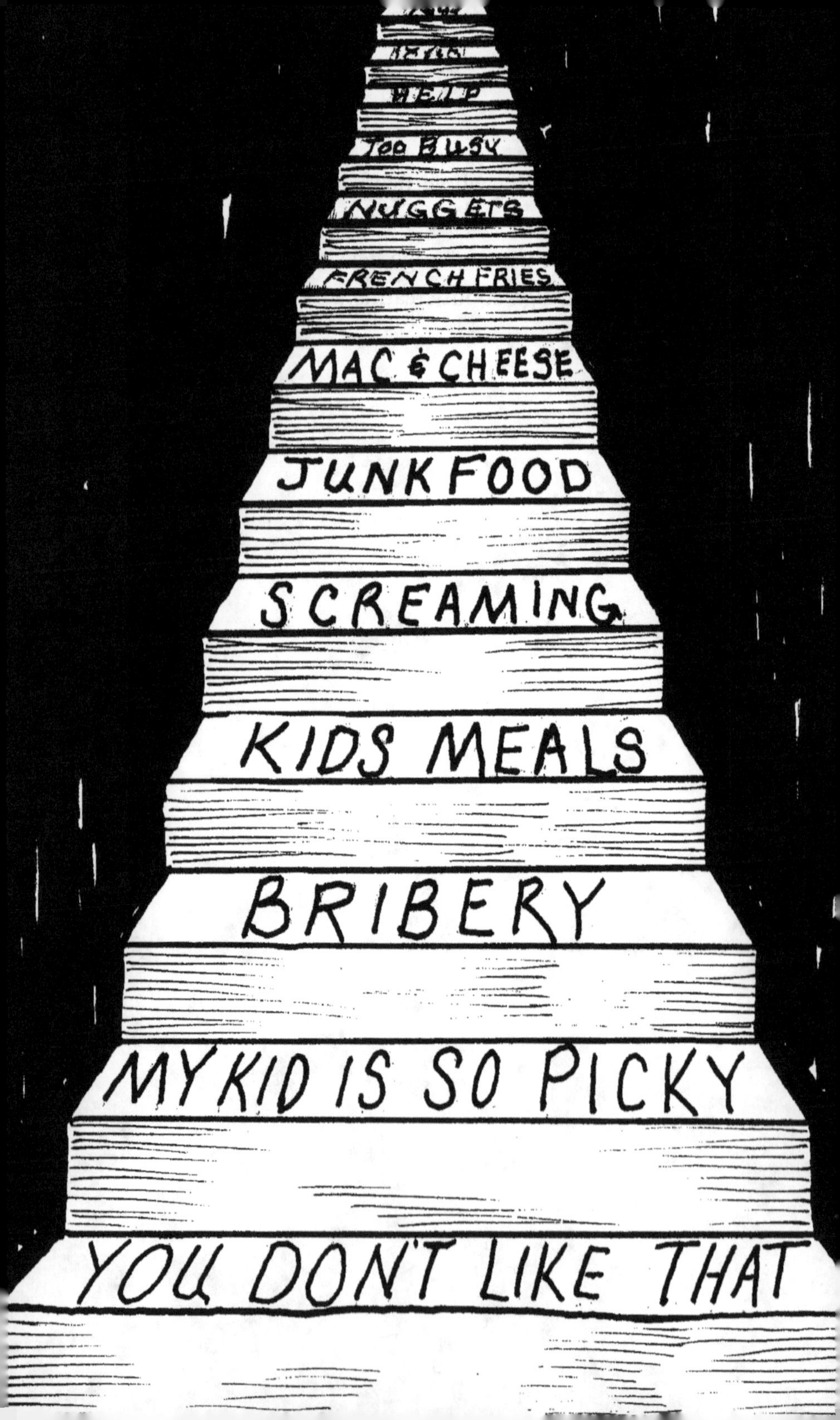

TOO BUSY
NUGGETS
FRENCH FRIES
MAC & CHEESE
JUNK FOOD
SCREAMING
KIDS MEALS
BRIBERY
MY KID IS SO PICKY
YOU DON'T LIKE THAT

How to Create a Picky Eater in 15 Simple Steps

This section pokes some fun at how our society is creating a nation of picky eaters. Sometimes clarity comes from looking at a problem head-on, so let's tackle picky eating with a little humor. These are the behaviors and tactics that will take you in the opposite direction from where you want to go. If you gave birth to a child with sensitive taste buds today, and you followed these simple steps, you'd have a picky eater in no time!

Got a picky eater in your family? See if any of these behaviors ring a bell:

1. Picky Eater Reminders! Tell them they're picky.

A great way to create a picky eater is to make sure you remind your child when they are about to taste something or order something from a menu at a restaurant that...

"Honey, you don't like that."

"Sweetheart, that has peas in it."

"Michael, you don't like carrots."

"The last time you had one of those you spit it out!"

"You've never liked broccoli."

Kids' tastes change faster than the weather, so if your child says that they don't like something, respect them, but don't think for a second that it's a permanent state. Just keep offering them a wide variety of healthy foods including the one you think they'll never like in a million years, even the ones *you* think are disgusting. Just don't let them know you think that. You'll find yourself amazed at how, all of a sudden, they just start eating a food they've always disliked. And when I say "all of a sudden," I mean it could take years. That's right, it can take years for them to develop a taste for a new food. Just take your time (and more than a few deep breaths). You don't have to do all of your food parenting in one meal—that's why we have 18 years to raise them.

2. Within Earshot! Tell others they're picky.

Make sure when your child is in earshot you tell other people that....

"She won't eat that."

"He doesn't like those."

"She won't eat anything."

"He's my picky eater."

"She got my sweet tooth."

Kids believe what you tell them and what they hear you telling others. You have to believe that it is perfectly natural for your child to love healthy foods if you want them to actually love healthy foods. Many parents are skeptical of this, so all I can ask is that you try it. Even if you don't like spinach, keep offering it to them.

3. Feed them these 3 things...over and over and over. Chicken Nuggets, Mac & Cheese and Hot Dogs.

Feed your child the same foods over and over—hot dogs, chicken nuggets, and mac & cheese are all good choices. They are bland, so they won't exercise your child's taste buds. Since they are processed foods, they are made primarily from the same two ingredients anyway—corn and soy—and they are chemically designed to tap the same addictive centers in your brain as drugs, so that your child won't want to eat anything else.

Parents of very young children come to me all the time and tell me their child will only eat hot dogs or chicken nuggets. They've tried and tried and that is all they'll eat. To which I gently reply, "At six years old, where are they getting all these hot dogs?" "Who is buying them the chicken nuggets?" Especially when your kids are young, *you* get to decide what goes in the grocery cart and their mouth.

Your child may be unhappy, but he's not going to die or end up malnourished if you cut off his supply of nuggets. He'll certainly end up malnourished if all he eats is a chicken nuggets lunch for the next twelve years of his life.

Trust me, if they're hungry they'll eat what you've made for dinner. It's ok for kids to be hungry at dinner, being hungry is what makes new foods taste good! Which brings us to our next trick for creating a picky eater.

4. Make Everyone in the Family a Different Dinner!

Instead of making one well-balanced meal, make each person in the family something different, something you know they will like. This way they don't have to try anything new and as an added bonus: you'll learn to hate cooking. Even better, if you have two or three picky eaters who all like different things, by all means make all of them separate meals – that's what micro-waves are for!

Families used to sit down to one meal where everybody ate the same thing. It was balanced with several items to choose from; a salad, green beans, boiled potatoes, a piece of grilled chicken. Now kids tell parents what they want to eat, not the other way around. Who's running this show anyway? It's time to take your parenting rights back! You get to decide what's for dinner, and your children will enjoy it once they know that's just the way dinner works. As I often tell my kids, nobody gets their favorite dinner every night, not even Mom.

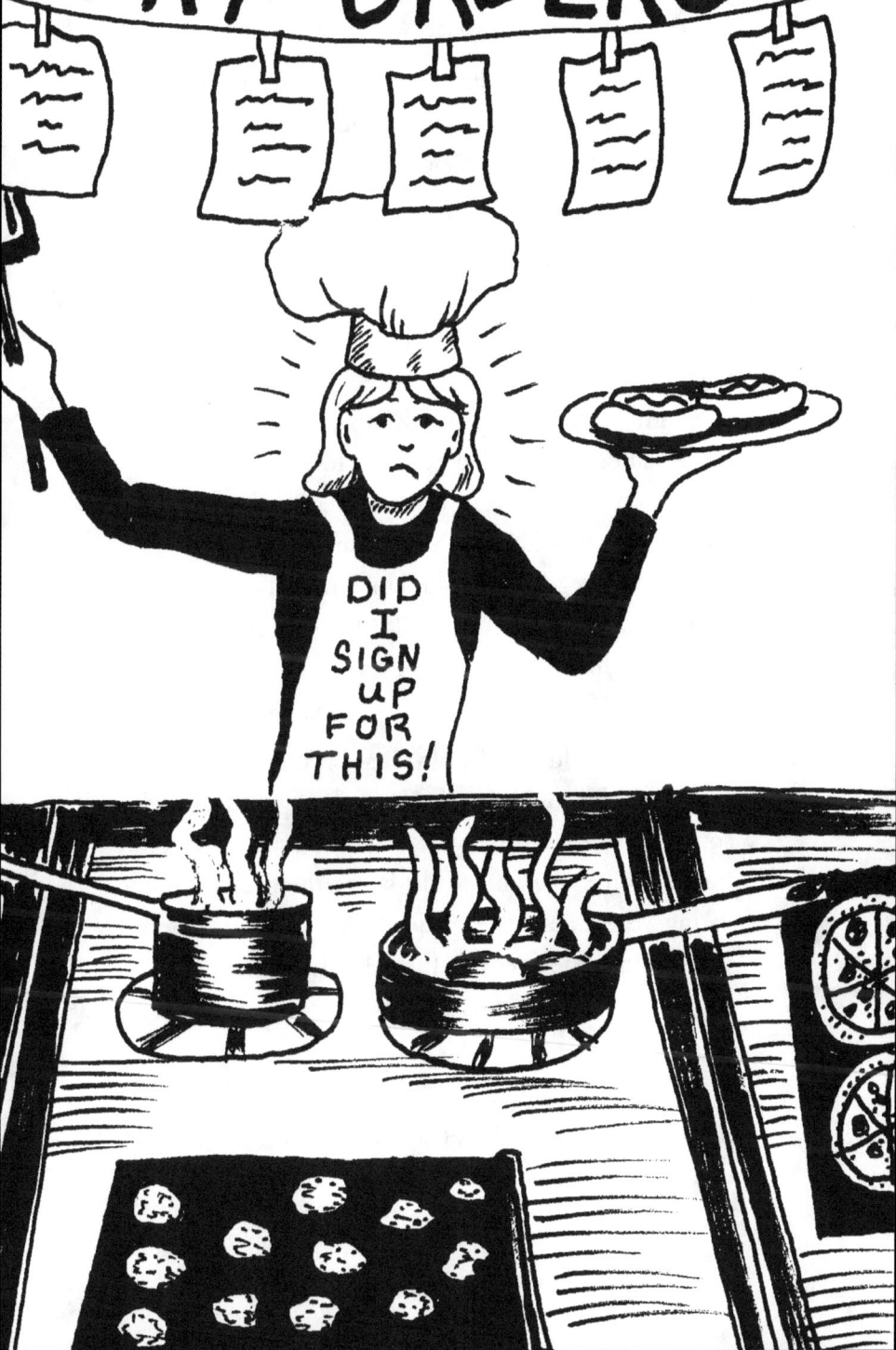

5. Pack them a lunch you know they'll eat. Be Consistent!

A great trick for developing a picky eater is to always pack the same items in your child's school lunch; it's fast, easy and you know she'll eat it!

Lunches are a hard nut to crack. You're not around to encourage them, there are all kinds of distractions and pressure from other kids, and they don't get much time to eat. So you have to get your child's buy-in about what foods they'll eat. What works will vary from child to child, but there are two things your child needs to understand. One is that wasting food costs the family money, so they need to be honest with you about what they will and won't eat at lunch. Two, they need to eat some vegetables at lunch. This is a difficult step though, so help your child find a combination that works for them.

Maybe four carrot sticks is too many. Could they eat one or two at lunch? Could they eat one or two sugar snap peas? Throw in a sliced raw beet or turnip with some dip. One or two bites might not seem like a lot, but all you are trying to do is get them comfortable eating vegetables—the quantity doesn't matter at this point. Once they get comfortable, they'll have the rest of their life to eat them!

6. Reward them for eating vegetables!

This is probably my favorite way to create a picky eater...reward your child for eating vegetables with ice cream, cake or candy. You know what I mean. At the end of the day it's just easier to bribe your child to eat healthfully. "If you eat all your vegetables you can have a cupcake!" "Two more bites of broccoli and you can have some ice cream!" This is a sure-fire trick to creating a picky eater.

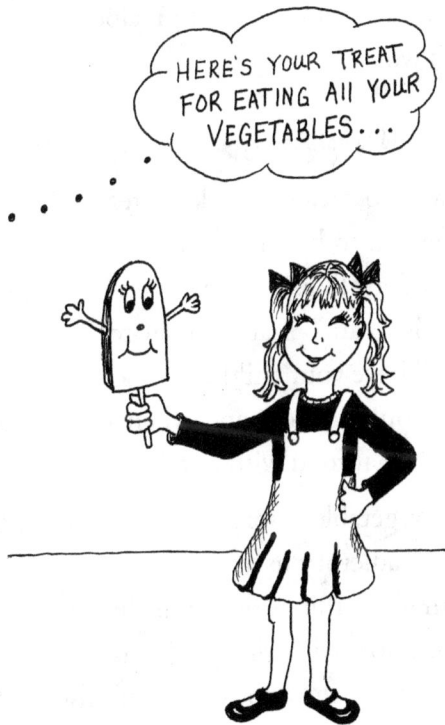

Every time you do this you're sending the opposite message you want your child to receive. Basically, you're telling them that vegetables taste so bad you have to be rewarded if you eat them. This is one of the places where you need to examine your own beliefs. It takes time, but you both can learn to see vegetables as delicious. Look at it this way…desserts are good but often are not good for you. Vegetables are good (when fixed properly), and they are good for you. So don't accidently send your kids the wrong message. There are thousands of ways to fix broccoli. If you don't like broccoli, you just haven't found the right recipe yet! (Luckily for you, that's what Pinterest is for!)

7. Force your child to eat their vegetables. "Eat it or Else!"

A great way to create a picky eater and a child that has an aversion to healthy food is to force them to eat things they don't like. "You're not leaving the table until your plate is clean." "Eat your broccoli Michael, every bite." You'll have your children choking and gagging all the way through dinner and when they're adults they won't touch that food with a ten foot pole.

Kids need vegetables more than any other food group, but as contradictory as it sounds, you don't want to force them to eat things they don't like. It creates a negative association with the food, makes mealtime unpleasant, and has the opposite effect of what you want.

8. Buy your child a "Kids Meal" when you go out to eat.

If you're really having trouble creating a picky eater, just buy your child a kids' meal whenever you eat at a restaurant. They're cheap and you know they'll eat them because kids' meals are pretty much the same everywhere you go—pink slime-filled burgers, not-chicken nuggets, unnatural orange mac & cheese, and who-knows-what's-inside those hot dogs. They're pretty much made of the same three ingredients: chemicals, corn and soy.

Kids' meals are nutritionally a big ZERO. They lack vitamins, minerals, phytonutrients, antioxidants, enzymes, and fiber. They are usually fried, filled with chemical preservatives, artificial colors and flavors, bad fats like hydrogenated and partially hydrogenated oils, and a host of other lord-knows-what ingredients. So where's the bargain in that, for you or your kids?

9. If they scream really loud or throw a fit, give them a cookie to keep the peace.

A great way to raise a picky eater is to avoid conflict at mealtime by only feeding your child things they like to eat. It's the end of the day, you're tired, they're tired, and who wants a scene at TGI Fridays with all those judgmental yuppies without kids gawking at you! Picky eaters love this trick. I think they strategically position their screams for when the yuppies are about to sip their martinis.

Here's the best parenting tip I can give you: don't ever give in to your child when they scream or throw a fit. Trust me, you'll regret it for the next 18 years. If your child starts to scream, your best bet in the long run and in the moment is to pick them up and take them outside or to the car. You do this once or twice and you'll probably never have to do it again. Your child will know that this isn't the way to get what they want. This is not about punishing your child, it's about removing them from the situation, when they are acting inappropriately.

10. Quick and easy is the key to picky.

If you want to raise a picky eater, feed them lots of convenience foods. They're quick to prepare and the food companies designed them to appeal to the sugar, salt, and fat receptors in the brain, so your kids are sure to like them. This will also help train their taste buds to expect lots of sugar, salt, and fat in their meal. They likely won't find real food very appealing anymore.

The problem with processed convenience foods is that they truly do alter your child's taste buds, since they're actually designed in a laboratory to be ultra-appealing and to tap the same centers in the brain as addictive substances like nicotine and cocaine.

Fresh fruit doesn't taste sweet if your child has been eating candy or cookies throughout the day, and vegetables don't taste as good if you're eating potato chips and French fries with every meal. Even if you can't stick to this rule all the time, try and save the junk food for a once-in-a-while treat after a nice meal or on weekends. You'll be amazed that your kids actually learn to eat based on what you regularly feed them.

11. Employ the Picky Eater Pre-Meal Meal Strategy.

Parents who are really serious about creating a picky eater have a unique pre-meal strategy that virtually guarantees they'll wind up with a picky eater. On their way to a friend's house for dinner, if they're afraid the friend might make something unusual or something their child might not like, they stop on the way and get them a Happy Meal® to eat before they arrive. This strategy ensures your child never has to try anything new. Works every time.

This approach teaches your child that new foods are scary, when the opposite is true. They may not like every new food they try, but a world of wonderful foods with immune boosting nutrients opens up to them when they try new foods on a regular basis. If they express concern about eating at a friend's house, just let them know they don't have to eat anything they don't care for; they just need to taste everything they are being served. Remember, it's actually a good thing for your child to get hungry; they'll appreciate food more and it will taste better.

12. Order your kids French fries every time you go out to eat. French Fries Please!

Step number 12 for creating a picky eater…Always order your kids French-fries when you're out at a restaurant. They'll fill up on these awesome little treats, and the excessive salt and fat will make any healthy food you get them seem like nothing worth eating. And an added bonus…you can eat some of their French fries without having to feel guilty about ordering your own!

Ok, ok…I know French fries are amazing, and a life without French fries is truly a life not worth living, but that doesn't mean you have to order them every single time you go out to eat. The one thing you should get in the habit of ordering, every time you go out to eat, is a salad. This is one of your secret weapons for getting your family to eat their vegetables. So skip that basket of free bread and instead order everyone in the family a beautiful green salad before you even place your order. This is truly a priceless tip, so give it a try. Even if they don't like salad, or they say they don't want one, watch what happens when the waitress sets one down in front of everyone in the family while they wait for their dinner. Even kids who don't like salad will eventually eat it because….well…there's nothing better to do. You might have to order them salads a number of times before they'll eat it, but if it means you'll eventually raise a child who enjoys a pre-meal salad for the rest of their life it will be some of the best money you've ever spent! If you're worried about wasting food, just order two salads and 4 plates. Then give everyone at the table a smaller serving of salad.

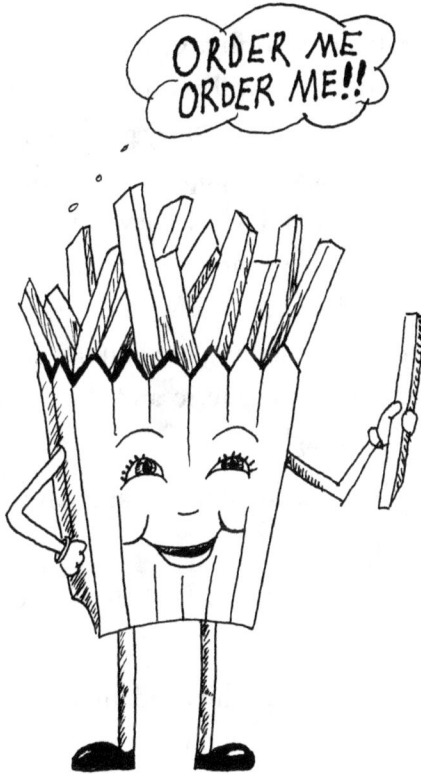

13. Don't get your child involved in meal planning or preparation unless it's...."Michael, Come set the Table."

Picky eaters typically see meal time as boring, so a great way to promote the picky eater mindset is to give your child the same job every night, such as setting the table, because you know it's what they can handle. Whatever you do, don't let them help with any kind of food preparation. Just think of the mess they are likely to make!

Setting the table is boring. Get your kids engaged in meal preparation; this will get them excited about new foods. Right before dinner they're likely to be hungry so they're also likely to pop whatever they're preparing into their mouth. Presto! They just tried something new without even knowing it and without you asking. If not every night, then start with once in a while, and make meal prep something fun you do with your kids. Put on some jammin' music and do a little dancing with your chopping!

NOTE: Helping make dinner is also advantageous for these reasons:

a. It teaches them how to feed themselves, a lost art these days.

b. It gives them ownership and they're likely to feel proud of their contribution to the meal and thus more likely to eat it.

c. It teaches them how much time and energy it takes to prepare a healthy meal so they'll be more appreciative the next time you make them something.

There are many things even small hands can do. Most kids love peeling carrots or shredding cheese. We have an egg slicer that we use to slice mushrooms or peeled kiwi that made my kids squeal with delight when they were younger. (Even now as teenagers, they still get a kick out of using it.) And the piece de' resistance in our kitchen? A Pampered Chef food chopper. It's like free therapy. A few whacks at the ol' food chopper not only chops walnuts, apples and celery down to perfect waldorf salad size, but gets rid of all of the days' frustrations.

14. Feed them grab and go breakfasts because mornings are hard.

With the crazy packed lives we all lead, you really need a grab and go breakfast or you're likely to head out the door with nothing to eat at all. And feeding your kids sugary cereals or "breakfast bars" instead of real food is also a great way to raise a picky eater. They're fast and fun and companies put so many "vitamins" in them that they're likely bursting with healthy. (Besides, that tiger, rabbit, and leprechaun are so darn cute!)

When you feed your child a sweetened boxed cereal for breakfast you're basically serving them a bowl of sugar with some vitamins thrown in. Cereal companies will try and hide the sugar by calling it names you can't pronounce, but it's in there, and if you added all of the different types of sugar together it would most likely be the first and most prominent ingredient. So save the boxed cereal and cereal bars for a treat after a meal and feed your child real food for breakfast: eggs, oatmeal with bananas and cinnamon, a bagel with peanut butter or cream cheese, or even some left-overs or soup are all wonderful options. Want something really quick? Make up some little snack bags of raisins and walnuts, something with real power to build up the brain cells and their immune system.

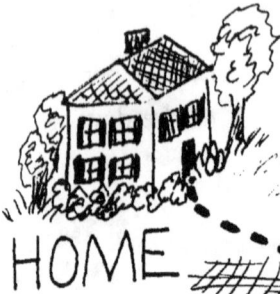

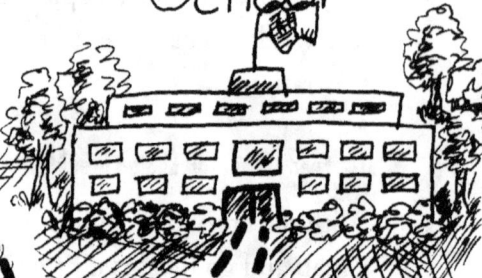

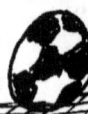

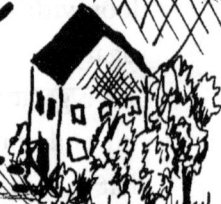

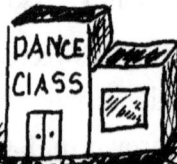

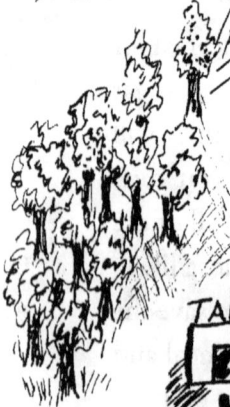

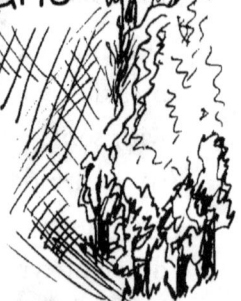

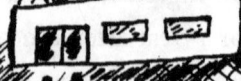

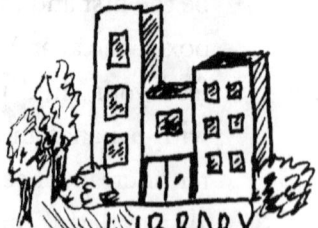

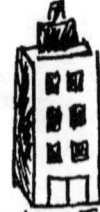

15. Over Schedule Your Life.

Schedule so many extracurricular activities that you don't have time to sit down and eat, much less make dinner. Picky eaters love this lifestyle because it means they get to pick which microwave dinner or fast food restaurant meal they are going to eat each night. They usually get the same thing too, over and over and over.

Extracurricular activities are important, but too many things scheduled during the week means the family dinner goes out the window. Each family needs to make their own choices when it comes to scheduling their week, but keep in mind there's a lot of magic that happens around the family dinner table. You may not feel it at one meal, but over the years it's where your kids really get to know you, themselves and each other.

Dinner at home is a completely different experience than dinner at a restaurant. Eating at home is quiet. A home cooked meal means a relaxed time together where your kids can share with you the events of their day and the challenges they are facing without a waitress interrupting every few minutes or a television (or six) blaring in the background. It's where you teach your children what foods nourish their bodies. It doesn't have to be every night, but make sure the family dinner doesn't get the shaft as you race through your life. It's one of your most valuable parenting tools.

So, do you think it's worthwhile to put some time and energy into raising a child who isn't afraid to eat over at a friend's house and enjoys eating healthy food? Do you think you're ready for fewer mealtime battles and no more making different meals for different kids? If so, you'll enjoy this next section. It takes you inside the mind of a picky eater and gives you lots of tips, tricks, and strategies for raising kids who eat a diverse diet of whole foods.

There's an added bonus too! These same strategies will also help you build a stronger relationship with your kids, stronger family bonds, and happier, healthier, well-adjusted kids. It's a win-win all the way around and it's fun and easy. (Well, easy-ish!)

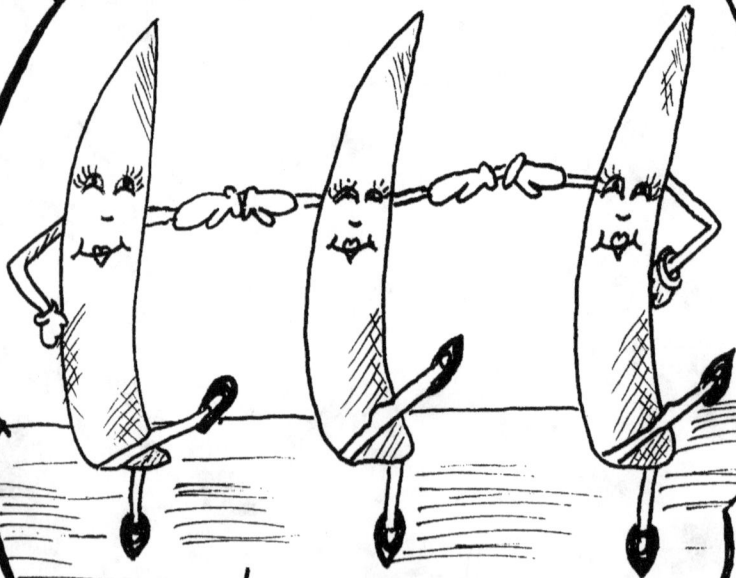

How to Raise a Child who Loves Healthy Food

NOTE: Don't try and tackle all of these at once. Pick what you can reasonably handle, achieve success, and pick something else to tackle in the next round.

Rule # 1: Enjoy Yourselves!

Above everything else, make eating healthfully a pleasant experience. This can be a challenge for the parent of a picky eater because they often find it hard to believe a child will develop a taste for healthy foods. It takes time, but remember, you've got 18 years. It might seem crazy....but your only job when it comes to eating healthfully is to teach them that it's fun and enjoyable. This means you have to believe it yourself. (You do believe it don't you? Of course you do!) It may be a direct challenge to the way you were raised or to your experience as a child, but if you don't believe vegetables really taste good, your child never will.

Rule #2: Give a Poor Vegetable a Chance

There are literally thousands of ways to prepare each vegetable. I'd argue that it's difficult to say you don't like spinach. You probably just haven't found a recipe that connects with you yet, or you haven't given it enough tries. Most people give up trying a food way before their body is capable of developing a taste for it, and I know lots of picky eaters that have never even tried the foods they say they don't like. Crazy, right?

You may need to re-train your taste buds with your child. Remember, it could take years before you develop a taste for a new food. But you're not going to give up after only 15 tries are you? Fifteen tries is for quitters. And you are no quitter. (The mere fact that you are still reading this book and haven't thrown your e-reader against the wall is evidence of that!)

I've seen it take years for a picky eater to warm up to a new food, but think about it: if it takes your child five years to develop a taste for broccoli, that means that they're likely to have 80-90 years of eating broccoli over the course of their life. There's a boatload of antioxidants in 80 years of immune-boosting broccoli!

So if you don't like steamed broccoli, maybe try sautéing it with some extra virgin olive oil and garlic. Not a fan of green beans? Try stir-frying them in a tiny bit of butter and soy sauce...now that's addictive!

And if even ranch dressing or hummus won't get you to eat your carrots (what are you, crazy?), try roasting them with some honey and slivered almonds. (And if you really want to go wild, toss in some crumbled goat cheese and cranberries after they come out of the oven—the explosion of flavor will make you weep tears of joy.) Branch out, live a little, live dangerously if you have to, but get out there and try some new recipes!

Rule # 3: No Force Necessary

Don't force your child to eat things they don't like.

If they don't like something, the trick is not to make a big deal out of it: just have them taste it and move on to talking about your day. Then the next day, a few weeks or months later, whatever feels right, set a snack plate next to them while they are watching TV or playing a video game with a bite or two of that food on the plate. Keep doing this over and over. It just takes time. And don't be surprised if one day they start popping fresh snap peas in their mouths from the snack plate you laid on the table.

(Whatever you do, do not start doing the happy dance and exclaim, "I told you snap peas were delicious!" They will certainly stop eating them immediately just to spite you if you do that.)

Rule #4: Tiny Bite

Everyone in the family needs to at least taste everything on the plate. This is a very important rule: little tastes are fine, but everyone needs to try what's made

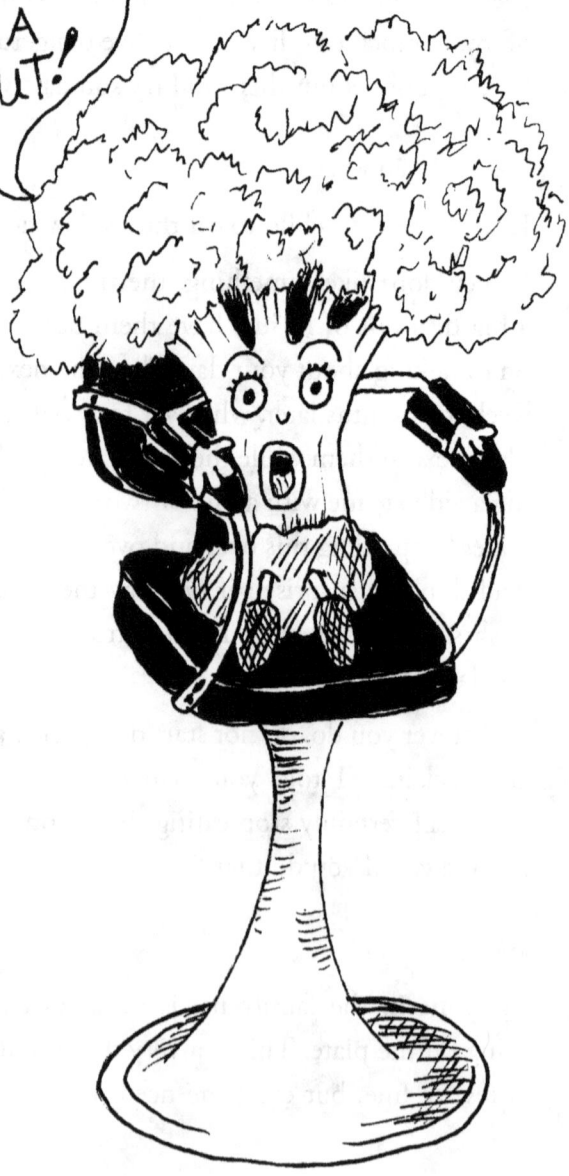

for dinner. If they don't care for it, no problem, there are usually two or three other things on the table that they can eat.

When my kids were small and didn't like what was being served, we used to have a "biggest tiny bite" contest and see who could take the biggest tiny bite. It didn't always work, but oftentimes the competitive nature of my children overrode the stubbornness of not wanting to eat even one tiny bite of something. Be creative without being condescending. Your kids will know if you're just trying to trick them and your heart isn't in it.

When they are little, teach your kids how to give broccoli hair cuts—just hold up the little broccoli floret and give him a trim with your teeth. They can give a Mohawk, a buzz or anything else they can think of. Kids just love this stuff. Make mealtime a time for creative exploration, relaxation, and connection with your family.

If they don't care for anything being served, you can always let your kids get something else healthy to eat after dinner, but they can't jump up and eat something else while dinner is going on. We have a rule at our house that you have to wait an hour before going back into the kitchen for food after dinner. In some families, it's thirty minutes. The most important thing is that they sit and enjoy dinner with the family even if they don't do more than taste what is being served.

The power of the family dinner is phenomenal for getting kids to eat healthfully, but your child has to appreciate that you put time and energy into preparing a healthy meal, so it's not ok for them to run off and eat something else.

What happens next? They get bored sitting there watching everyone else enjoy dinner. It's not a punishment or a power struggle…it's no big deal, this is just how we do dinner. Then, before you know it, they start nibbling at the wonderful assortment on their plate. Don't say a word. Just keep on enjoying your meal and your beautiful family.

Rule #5: Understand the Meaning of Dinner

We've kind of lost sight of what it means to have dinner. The media creates an idealized, unrealistic vision of dinnertime as this perfect experience where no one is belching or spilling their milk and all the kids are getting along just fine. That's not dinner for most people. In fact, dinner is hardly ever perfect. It is a powerful parenting tool, however, so don't underestimate it. You won't see the effects at one meal, but you'll see dramatic effects over the course of their life.

Dinner is…

Everyone sitting down to the table at the same time in the evening to enjoy some food and talk about their day.

It's preparing and sharing one meal together as a family. Someone making the salad, someone else sautéing the vegetables, grilling the meat, or slicing the bread. The time spent preparing the meal is time that builds your relationship with your children. So put on some music, tell some jokes, let them experiment with the sautéed vegetables, and above all enjoy each other's company.

It's the number one place where kids learn what foods they should be eating to sustain their bodies.

It's how your children will learn how to make a healthy meal and a nice salad for themselves and their families! It's a special time and space in our busy lives where family relationships are built, challenges are overcome, funny stories are told, and if all goes as planned, perhaps a vegetable or two is consumed.

I get it—we all have busy lives. Sports, after-school activities, mom's night out at the local wine bar, are all things that occasionally get in the way. There are nights that the thought of dinner makes me cringe! That's ok too. The point is making an effort to make this the exception rather than the rule.

Rule #6: 1-Hour Barrier

No eating one hour before or after dinner. Food tastes so much better when you are hungry, so let your children come to the dinner table ready to eat. If they really can't wait, give them raw vegetables to munch on like green beans, sugar snap peas, carrot sticks or sliced cucumber…things that won't spoil their appetite. This is another place where you might want to examine your own beliefs about food. It's okay to be hungry. Humans can survive at least 21 days without food. (I'm not suggesting this of course, but it would be one way to get your kid to eat his vegetables!)

What gets people into trouble is the blood sugar crashes that come from eating processed foods. With a blood sugar crash you don't just get hungry (that empty feeling in your stomach), you actually become

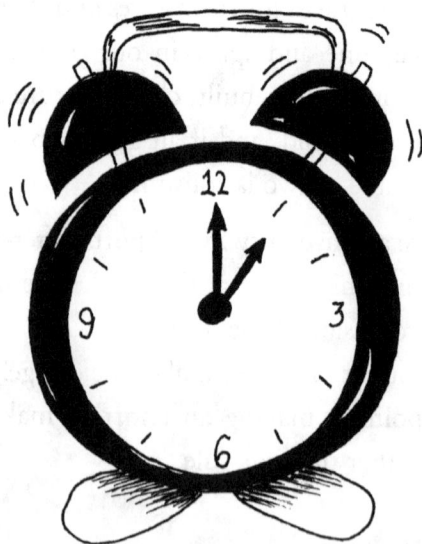

irritable and feel bad all over. For that situation, you need to get your kids a little protein: a little handful of raw nuts, a stick of string cheese or a small slice of turkey are all good choices. For the most part, being hungry is really a good thing. It gives your digestive system a much-needed rest and it makes healthy food taste wonderful.

Rule # 7: Meaningful Rewards

Reward your kids with hugs, notes, time with you, or a story, not candy.

You may say, "Jeez, what's wrong with rewarding your child with a lollypop?" If that was the only candy or sweet treat they'd had that day, or that week, it might not be a problem. The problem today is that kids are fed sugar at every turn: their breakfast is often loaded with sugar, teachers are handing out candy, after-school snacks and soccer practice sweets are filled with sugar. So that lollypop? It's just the chemically-induced cherry on top of an already sugar-filled day.

Our 4th of July parade used to be filled with homemade floats pulled by lawn mowers, cars or tractors. Now people just fill up grocery carts with candy and throw it at the kids along the parade route. No one seems to notice that the kids aren't watching the clowns in mini cars anymore - they're all racing around and wrestling each other to the ground for the mass of candy strewn about.

There are all kinds of ways you can reward yourself and your kids, so give some thought to what you are teaching them with your choice of rewards.

Your body can handle a certain amount of sweet treats, but make sure they aren't the primary tools in your rewards arsenal. As you give your children rewards, you are in effect teaching them how to take care of themselves. Why not give them a wide array of wonderful choices? Why not make the majority of the rewards be both good and good for them? That way when they are 35 and stressed at work, they come home to a good book instead of reaching for an ice cream cone.

The Magic of a Good Book: A trip to the bookstore is an excellent choice for rewarding your child. You can teach them how to browse an online book store, take a trip to a used book store or one of the larger new book stores with a café and a whole section cordoned off for children filled with little tables, chairs, fake trees, puppets and every children's book you could imagine. Or spend the day at an antique bookshop. In our city, we have an antique bookshop downtown that is four beautiful stories high with dramatic wooden floors, aisles and aisles of books, and windows that go from the floor to the ceiling looking out over the city.

When you take your child to the bookstore, you teach them to reward themselves with something that doesn't put pounds on their body or stress on their heart. Instead, you open up an endless world of adventure. Don't have time to go to the bookstore? Take them on a virtual tour of Amazon's bookstore and let them get a package in the mail. They can even watch the tracking as the package gets closer to the house.

And let's not forget our public library. Rewarding your child with a trip to the library not only rewards them with the wonder of books, it teaches them how to be responsible citizens by treating their borrowed books gently and returning them on time.

Whether you're buying or borrowing, a book is definitely a reward that's both good and good for you.

The Power of a Simple Note: Take a moment and write your child a personal note or letter. Many people think kids will prefer candy over everything else, but a lot of that is taught behavior—that's just what they're used to and the sweet taste makes them feel good in the short run. A card hidden under their pillow is much more powerful, and just as easy, while the impression can last a lifetime.

I have a friend who has a little mailbox outside her daughter's bedroom and regularly sends her "mail" as a reward for good deeds or just a simple "I love you." Her daughter is graduating high school this year and the mailbox is still there. My friend tells me that sometimes her daughter rolls her eyes now when she receives a note congratulating her on a good grade or good deed, but then she puts the note in a special box with all the other notes my friend has written her over the years. (She may pretend she's outgrown it, but I don't think she'd keep the mailbox outside her door and save her notes if she had.)

The more specific you are in the note the better. Saying "I'm proud of you" is nice, but saying "I'm proud of the great job you did helping your grandmother with her flower bed. It's just beautiful. You have a strong artistic eye" is much more impactful. They'll likely keep that note the rest of their lives, if not in its physical form, then in their mind and in the boost that it gives to their self-esteem.

Say it with words: You don't have to write it down though. Don't underestimate the power of the spoken word either. Teach your children that when you say "I'm proud of you" it's a big deal. Watch your child throughout the day developing the habit of acknowledging their successes and positive behavior. Don't assume an ice cream cone is a better reward than a simple "nice job today."

The Power of a Game: Play a game with your kids. We have so many things on our mind and our to-do lists we often feel we don't have the time (or patience) to push little plastic pieces around a board all afternoon.

But, here's the secret… Playing a box game is not really about the game; it's about the conversations you get to have with your child while you play. Parents often wish their teens would talk to them more. Playing games with them is a great way to help your child develop the habit of talking to you, confiding in you about things that are on their mind, asking questions about life. It may not happen every game, but over the years you'll be surprised what you can learn about your child in a

30-60 minute game. Most importantly, you want to create the opportunities for those conversations to take place.

Finally, when you play a game with your child as a reward, you are teaching them how to reward themselves with something that's good for their mind and their health.

Night out on the Town: One of my favorite rewards was to take the kids to a nice restaurant for dinner. This is not just a treat, but a wonderful education about the art and beauty of food. Make it an adventure! Let them taste what's on your plate and give their dish a try. Talk with them about what the different ingredients or spices might be and ask the chef to come to the table if you have specific questions and it's not too busy. It can be expensive to eat at a nice restaurant, but consider the richness of the experience not just of the food. One-on-one time with your child is priceless even if you only get to do it once or twice when they are young. It will be an evening they will remember the rest of their life.

So be creative and don't just resort to a lollypop or ice cream as a treat. Make it a treat to tell them a story when you get in the car. If you're not a storyteller, try telling a story together. We get everyone in the car creating one GIANT story. The crazy twists and turns each person brings to the story always result in laughter and a good time.

If you like to actually give them a little treat once in a while, instead of candy, try keeping a few inexpensive little toys in your purse or in a drawer at home. These will often keep them occupied for the car ride home longer than a piece of candy, and they won't ruin the taste of the fresh peaches or grapes you just purchased at the market!

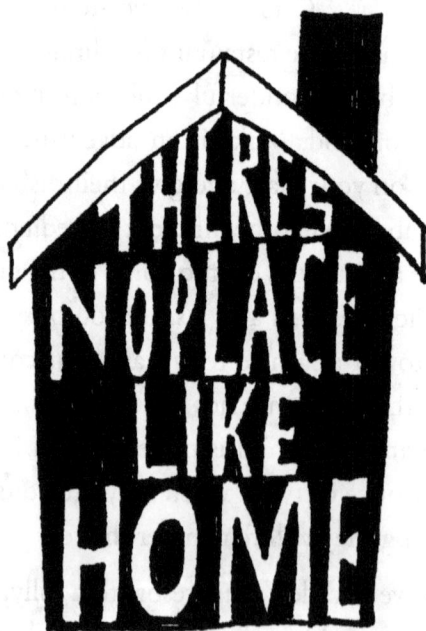

Rule # 8: Eat at home

There are endless reasons to eat at home, even though we live in a world where it is increasingly difficult to do so. Late nights at work, after school activities, empty refrigerators, and a lack of creative energy all make preparing a meal at the end of the day nearly impossible. However, studies show that kids who eat at home are healthier, get better grades and are happier. There is something sustaining about sitting around the dinner table: it gives your family the space it needs to build and rekindle relationships. The challenge is, you often can't see the effects at an individual meal. An individual meal can make you want to pull your hair out or join the traveling circus that's passing through town! With all the whining, the mess, and the kids fighting, an individual dinner can sometimes feel like a masochistic endeavor. Why would you put yourself through that?

Why eating at home is one of the best parenting tools you'll have in your parenting toolbox:

Meaningful Time With Your Kids: Don't worry if an individual dinner isn't perfect. Focus instead on how you deal with the imperfections that come with every dinner you make. This may sound crazy, but it is in those imperfections that you'll learn how to relate to your children in a meaningful and enjoyable way. That sounds like a lot to ask from dinner, but keep in mind you've got 18 years to perfect the art of parenting, so don't try and get there all in one night.

No Mystery Ingredients: Eating at home can be a significant boost to your family's health simply because you'll be more likely to know what's going into the food, because you're the one who put it in there. Here are just a few examples:

Want to cut back on salt? The worst thing you can do is get rid of your salt shaker! Why? Because 80% of your salt is coming from processed foods. All getting rid of your salts shaker will do is make the food you make at home bland so you'll want to go out to eat!

Want to cut back on sugar? If you cut back on anything, you should cut back on your sugar intake, but most people think that means they have to give up desserts. That's not where the majority of sugar is coming from, according to Dr. Robert Lustig:

- 1/3rd is from sweetened beverages
- 1/2 is coming from processed foods!
- Only 1/6th is coming from desserts.

Eating more meals at home is so important that we've included a How to Eat at Home Guide at the end of this book to make it really easy for you. When I coach families about eating at home they expect it to be an additional chore in their already packed lives. Instead, they come back to me the next week amazed at how much fun it is to prepare meals together as a family and how much it brings the family together. They find it doesn't detract from their day—it often makes their day more enjoyable!

Rule # 9: Veggie Adventure

Make trying new foods an adventure—it's a great metaphor for life. The more things in life you enjoy, the more fun you'll have. However, you have to try things you might not like in order to find the gems you love. It's a little like flipping stones in a creek bed. You have to flip a few to find that salamander, but boy when you do find one, it's so exciting! Keep trying new things and you'll build up a treasure chest of foods you love.

A few adventures you can try…

Cash in Hand: When you go to the grocery, give your child five dollars and tell them they can buy anything they like, but it has to meet two criteria…

1. It must be something they've never tried before.

2. It has to be something that is good for them!

This is a great way to give them some freedom surrounding their food choices, but still teach them which foods are healthy, and that eating healthy foods can be fun. You can't just tell them you'll buy it for them, because that takes the fun out of it. Put the cash in their hot little hands and see what they come back with.

Any Recipe You Want: Let your child pick any recipe they've never tried before, and make it together. Laugh and giggle while you cook or put on some good music and let mistakes and messes happen without getting upset about them. The purpose is not a clean kitchen or a tasty dish, though you may wind up with both when you are done, it's to enjoy your child's company and have some fun together. These moments help build your child's positive relationship with food, and moments like this, spent with your child when they are young, are the ingredients for strong relationships when they are teenagers.

Restaurant Adventure: Instead of ordering one meal for each person, have your child order a number of new items off the menu that no one in the family has tried before. Make this a really special event, talk it up and get the whole family excited about it. Joke about possibly not liking anything you order before you get to the restaurant. You'll be amazed at the new and wonderful foods you'll add to your list of things you love to eat.

First Friday Adventure: Have the first Friday of the month (or maybe just one or two nights a year, like the first day of each season) be the night that you try a new recipe! Make a big deal out of it, buy some balloons, and rent a movie afterward, and make a night of it. Remember, nobody has to eat anything they don't like, but everyone in the family needs to give it at least a taste.

Food Museum: Take a field trip to a specialty food store. Go to a gourmet cheese shop and have the cheese monger share with you all about the different cheeses and where they are from. Have her give you some samples and let your child pick one to bring home to share with the rest of the family. Wander through an Asian or Indian grocery store and let your child pick a few items to try or just stop by the ethnic section of your local grocery store. Remember, you often have to try something new multiple times before you develop a taste for it.

⭐ Tastes good & good for you	Tastes good & bad for you
Tastes bad & bad for you	Tastes bad & good for you

Rule # 10: Teach your child that there are 4 kinds of food....

Over time, kids start to think that foods that taste good are bad for you and foods that taste bad are good for you. (Parents and the media do a great job of reinforcing this belief.) You need to let your child know that there are really 4 kinds of food. (See illustration) What goes in the quadrants will be different for each person.

All across the world, people have different food patterns. The trick is to teach your child that they get to decide what goes into each quadrant. Individual foods can move from quandrant to quandrant over time, but the more foods you can put in the good and good for you quandrant, the healthier you'll be.

How do you do that? By trying and retrying new foods that are good for you on a regular basis. That's the key to eating healthy—filling up your first quadrant with new things you like. When you do that you don't feel deprived, your life feels richer and being healthy becomes a pleasurable experience.

Make your own grid and talk to your picky eater about the importance of tasting new things so he can fill up his first quadrant! It will help your child to see that they have control over which foods they choose to put in that quadrant. As they try new foods, they can watch that first quadrant grow.

The younger you start, the better, but this works for adults as well as children, so you can start at any age. Just don't make yourself crazy by trying to tackle all of these strategies at once. The point is to understand the fundamentals outlined in this book and then chip away at them over time. Remember, it has to be an enjoyable experience for you and for your child or you won't keep moving forward. Now let's really have some fun! Check out some of the crazy things I've seen parents of picky eaters do over the years.

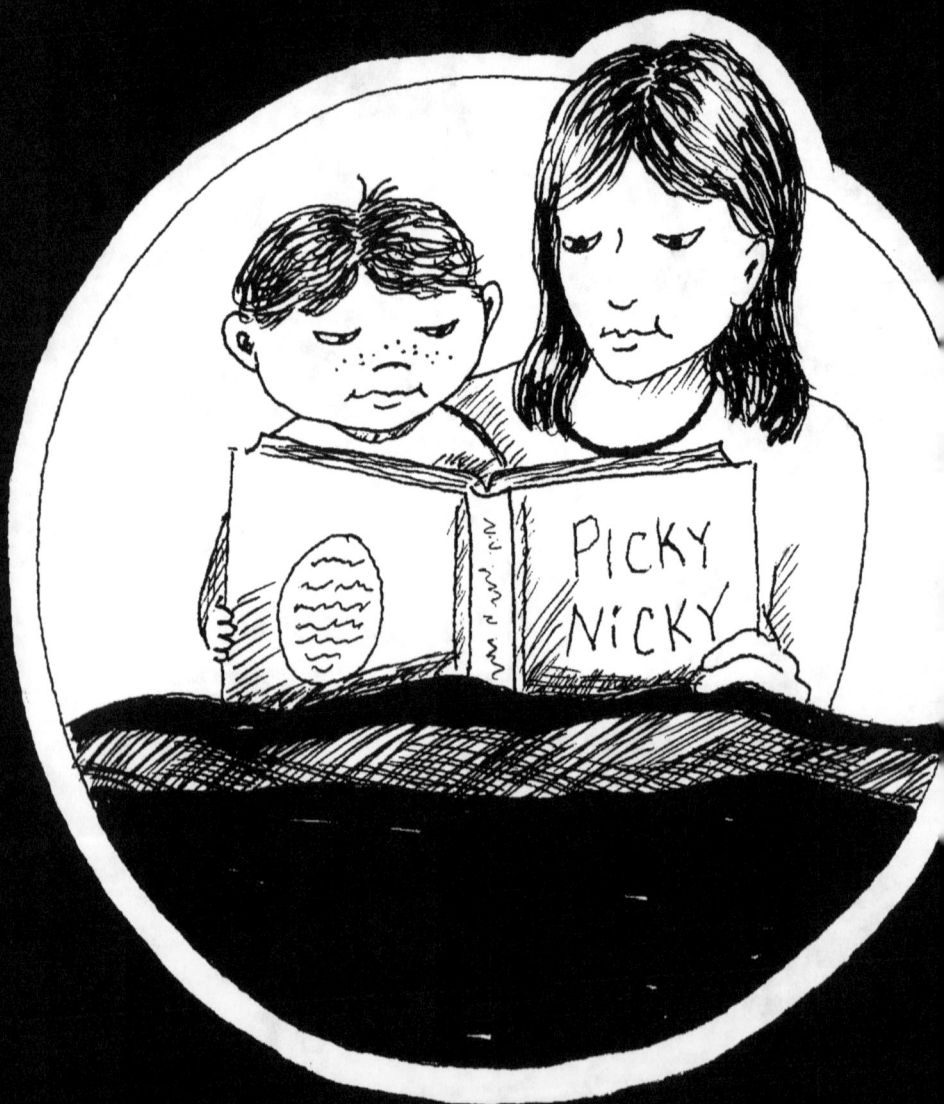

True Stories of Picky Eaters

If you have a picky eater in your family, and you probably do if you're reading this book, you might recognize one or two of the behaviors listed below. These are actual stories of picky eaters but the names have been changed to protect the (not so) innocent. What you say to your picky eater and what you believe about food will have a powerful impact on your child's perception of food.

Billy and Broccoli

When my son was two we had a play date with his friend Billy. I was making a bowl of steamed broccoli for a snack and I asked Billy's mother if she thought he would like some. She said, "No, he doesn't like broccoli." So I made my son a bowl and had it in my hand as I walked them to the door to leave. By the time Billy's mother and I had said goodbye, Billy had eaten the whole bowl of broccoli!

Annie and Kale

At another play date with my son's friend Annie, I made myself a scrambled-egg-and-sautéed-kale breakfast burrito. Now, regardless of what you might think of that combination, Annie was intrigued and asked if she could have some. Her mouth was open and she was about to take a bite when her mother stopped her and said, "Honey, you don't like kale." She stopped the bite inches from her mouth, and went off to play, never to eat kale again.

Michael and Chicken Nuggets

Michael's mom called me because her son had a poor diet, didn't like vegetables, and was about to get kicked off of the football team because of his weight. Michael went through our 30 Day Healthy Kids Fast Program. One afternoon, about halfway through the program, his mother picked him up from school. He was in tears because something bad had happened. In order to cheer him up, she offered to take him to McDonalds for his favorite, chicken nuggets. "No, Mom," he said, "I want you to take me home and make me some fish and a baked potato." That's a kid taking responsiblility for his own health.

Aaron and Papaya

I wanted my son to like papaya; it's at the top of the charts when it comes to nutrition, loaded with antioxidants, vitamins, and minerals. But papaya has a very strong taste, and he just didn't like it, even sprinkled with fresh lime which I find amazing. I offered it to him four to five times a year, for about 16 years. Then one afternoon while he was working intently at his computer, I brought him a small plate of fruit with one piece of papaya on it. As I handed him the plate I pointed to the papaya and said, "Aaron, please give this a try, it's so good for you." Then I left the room.

As I was walking out the door I noticed him pop the piece in his mouth. I was thankful, but didn't think too much of it. That evening, I had the rest of the papaya cut up on a plate during dinner. To my great surprise, he scooped a pile onto his plate and ate it! You might think 16 years is too long to try and get your kid to eat papaya, but he'll be enjoying both the nutrients and the taste of fresh papaya for the next 70 years!

Dad and Brussels Sprouts

I was coaching a family of five mostly to help with the youngest son who was an extremely picky eater. He'd had only chicken nuggets for lunch for the first seven years of his life. He wouldn't eat any fruits or vegetables and was reluctant to try anything new. As I was talking with the family about the most nutritious vegetables you can eat, the 15 super vegetables,* I came to Brussels sprouts. All of a sudden the father exclaimed, "no Brussels sprouts. That vegetable will never enter our house!"

Sounds like an adult who was forced to choke down Brussels sprouts as a child, doesn't it? I know a lot of people don't like Brussels sprouts. I spent the first 40 years of my life disliking them, but that statement made it very clear where their son was getting his "I won't taste anything" attitude. I, on the other hand, reluctantly give Brussels sprouts a try every now and then, and by now and then I mean once every couple of years, especially if someone puts a new recipe in front of me. At 40, to my great surprise, I've actually found a number of Brussels sprout recipes that I really like.

One was fried Brussels sprout leaves with a spicy dip at a trendy local restaurant on a trip to New England. My whole family liked them and it was one of the most enjoyable meals we've had as a family. So watch what you say about food—you don't have to eat anything you don't like—but try not to portray healthy foods as evil either.

Tommy and Nick and the Raw Turnip

I was at a company picnic a number of years ago and the host made a wonderful dip with sliced raw turnips. There were two little boys ages 6 and 8 who were both picky eaters. For dinner we were going to eat roast beef, carrots, and potatoes with gravy—nothing weird or unusual. Yet their mother had brought them hot dogs to eat because they didn't like roast beef, carrots or potatoes. As the meal was being prepared, the two boys were just gobbling up the homemade dip and raw turnips when their mother said… "Boys, that's enough. You'll spoil your dinner."

Aaaahhhhh! The horror of spoiling their nitrate and preservative filled hot dog dinner with the vitamin, mineral, phytonutrient and antioxidant filled raw turnips. Don't get me wrong, I love a good hotdog every now and then, but if your child would rather fill up on raw turnips let them go for it!

Hot dogs are for baseball games when your only other option is chemically induced liquid "cheese" nachos. (And pu-leaze don't say, "At least they have protein.")

Henry and The Hot Fudge Sundae

I was at our local ice cream parlor one afternoon and I saw a mom and dad with a three-year-old who they were harassing in order to get him to finish his ice cream. He was full and didn't want anymore…. "Come on Henry, you just have a few more bites." "Sit down and finish this." "Henry, take this," they said. as they shoved another bite in his mouth. Seriously? I'm sure they spent good money on that ice cream cone, and no one thinks wastefulness is good, but if they were able to take a step back and look at what they were doing, they would have laughed at the silliness of their behavior.

Practically everybody loves a good ice cream sundae, and life would be a lot less interesting without them, but one of the best lessons you can teach your child about eating healthy is to not use your body as a garbage disposal. If you go for a hot fudge sundae and you get to the last few bites and you're full, throw the rest out. Better to toss it than add it to their—or worse *your*—waist!

Brandon and The Bakery for Breakfast

This is one of my favorite parenting stories because it demonstrates so clearly how to create a child who screams when they don't get what they want to eat. I believe when your child cries, you should take it seriously. But crying about wanting a cookie isn't the same as crying because they are hurt or frightened.

One morning, a couple came into a bakery I worked at in New England with their three-year-old son. They were looking into the case with all the baked goods and asked their son what he wanted for breakfast. The son said "I want a cookie." The mother replied, "No, honey, it's breakfast time. You need to order a muffin." The son said, "No, I want a cookie!" They went back and forth a couple of times until the son started jumping up and down and screaming, "I want a cookie! I want a cookie!" So they bought him a cookie.

Perfect parenting behavior if you want your child to scream all of the time! If you don't want them to scream when they want a cookie, don't give them cookies if they scream. Instead, pick them up, take them out to the sidewalk or the car, and tell them they can go back in as soon as they stop screaming. Kids get bored really fast. For most kids, you only have to do this once, maybe twice, and they learn not to scream in public to get what they want. And while it's terrible while you're in the moment, it will pass. You have the strength inside you to wait out their temper tantrum, I promise!

The trick is to give your child a tool besides screaming, one that's polite and quiet but helps them get their point across. For my kids, I told them, "If you want something really badly, you don't have to scream. Just say 'Mom, I want this cookie really badly'" I explained that these are magic words and you can't use them all of the time or they loose their power. "Only use them when it really matters to you, and I'll try to respect that. It doesn't mean you'll always get what you want, but I'll know you want it really badly and I'll try and make it happen for you if I can." I made sure I honored that within reason, but they never got a cookie for screaming.

Sally and the School Lunch Programs

All over the country schools are attempting to change their lunch menus to include more healthy foods and finding that a lot of the real food is winding up in the trash.

In a local Washington D.C. school where they were having problems with kids throwing out the healthy things on their plate they tried a little experiment. One little girl in particular, we'll call her Sally, was throwing out her whole lunch. Then they started having a little new recipe taste test where kids got to vote on which recipe they liked the best. The winning recipe would then be featured on an upcoming menu. Low and behold even the pickiest kids started eating the new herbed carrots recipe. Even the little girl that had been throwing out her whole lunch found a new carrot recipe she liked!

We've spent 30 years teaching kids that they should be eating processed foods, let's put a little effort into getting them comfortable with and excited about the power of real food!

For more information on the exciting things that are happening in the school lunch programs across the country, check out the following links:

Lunch Lessons, Changing the Way we Feed Our Children - Ann Cooper at TEDxManhattan

https://www.youtube.com/watch?v=IVJv91n39Q8

Of Carrots and Kids: Healthy School Lunches that Don't Get Tossed - Dan Charles

http://www.npr.org/blogs/the-salt/2014/12/02/364712994/of-carrots-and-kids-healthy-school-lunches-that-dont-get-tossed

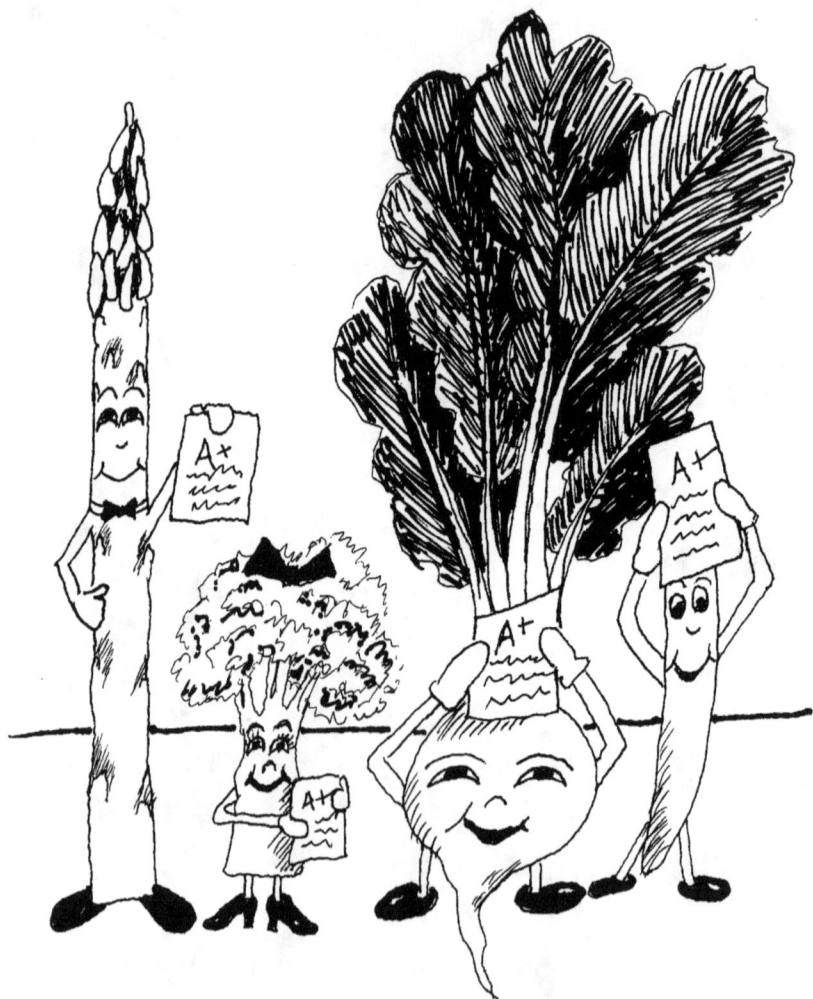

Super Vegetables

Super Vegetables: Not all vegetables are created equal. This list comes from the wonderful book Laurel's Kitchen, by Laurel Robertson. Think of these as the vegetables that get straight A's in nutrients!

- Asparagus
- Beet Greens
- Broccoli
- Brussels Sprouts
- Bok Choy
- Chard
- Collards
- Dandelion Greens
- Kale
- Mustard Greens
- Okra
- Sugar Snap Peas
- Snow Peas
- Spinach
- Turnip Greens

THINK BEFORE YOU SPEAK

The Power of Your Words

There are numerous tips, tricks and strategies in this book for helping you raise a child that loves healthy food. However, the single most important thing you can do, is to change your attitude toward food. You have to actually believe that eating healthy is more enjoyable than not eating healthy, that vegetables actually taste good, and that kids will not only eat them, but enjoy eating them. As you raise them you're helping to shape their worldview. Take a look at this example...

Racquetball with Toddlers!

I once took my sons, ages three and five, to the YMCA for the afternoon. As we passed the racquetball courts they became interested, so we got some racquets and went in to give it a try.

It was a disaster! We were only in there three minutes and racquets were flying everywhere. On each swing they were either hitting the ground or just missing a brother's head. In a panic, thinking one of them was about to lose an eye, I said, "ok guys... that's enough for today." I was about to add, "you guys are a little too young…We can try again when you're older." When my three-year-old cut me off and said, "Mom, wait till Dad hears how great we did!" I was about to tell them they weren't old enough to play racquetball and he thought they'd done great! Had the words gotten out of my mouth, you can bet he would have believed me. Instead, we left the court after three minutes and the boys felt like they were champions!

So pay attention to your own beliefs about eating, vegetables, and mealtime. There might be instances where you are creating or reinforcing the picky eater mindset.

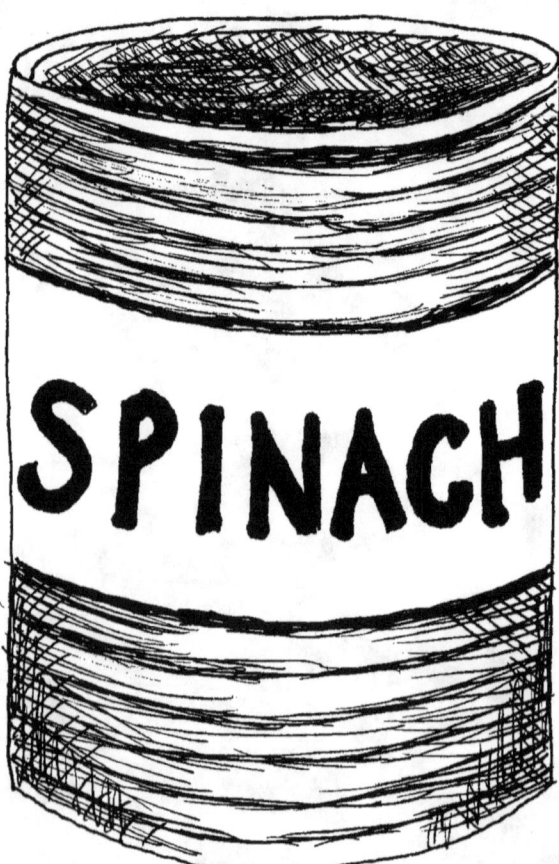

Where Did Popeye Go?

A lot of parents hope that their picky eater will just grow out of it, and for some picky eaters that's true. But there are two problems with the wait and see approach. One, they may not grow out of it. Two, it matters what your kids eat when they are young. That's when their bones and brains are developing. That's when they are laying the foundation for life-long eating habits. As parents, it's our job to give them the highest quality building materials we can so they can build strong bones, resilient minds, and a tough immune system.

If you're one of those people who doesn't believe kids will actually eat vegetables, think about this: kids all over the world eat vegetables and kids used to eat a lot more vegetables in this country than they do now. A balanced meal often gets the shaft with so much restaurant dining going on and convenience foods so readily available. But there's an additional problem that is driving the picky eater epidemic, and that's the power of the media. Food manufacturers want to sell parents and kids junk food because their profit margins are much higher on processed foods than whole foods. They spend billions of dollars trying to convince you and your kids that processed foods are good for you and that kids hate vegetables.

Quick Rule: If it says anything about being healthy on the package that's a good sign that it's not!

As my three-year-old son kicked back to watch Barney, a large purple dinosaur, sing and dance across the screen, a commercial came on with an adorable little cartoon girl sitting at a table with a plate of broccoli in front of her. Suddenly, the broccoli turned into a green monster and came off the plate at her! A look of horror came over her face, and then, some nice chewable candy vitamins came dancing across the screen and saved the day. What exactly are we teaching kids about food with this commercial? A lot of parents have started to believe that their kids won't eat vegetables, but that's not what we used to teach kids.

Where did Popeye the Sailor go? Let's overlook the fact that Olive Oil was oddly fickle and a bad role model for women, and focus on the fact that Popeye taught kids all over the world that spinach builds strong muscles. And he was right. He was our Super-Vegetable-Eating hero. Even kids who didn't really like spinach started eating it because they saw what it did for Popeye.

Childhood diabetes rates have tripled since the 70's, rare childhood cancers are up 400%, and we have an epidemic of autism, ADHD and childhood obesity.

Let's go back to teaching kids that vegetables are good for them! I say bring on the Broccoli Superheroes! Let them know that vegetables are their greatest defense against disease and their greatest resource for building strong bodies.

After the commercial break, my three-year-old son turned to me with a surprised but confident smile and said, "Mom look, Barney has a zipper!" Even very young kids are smart, smart enough to know that purple dinosaurs have zippers. And smart enough to understand that it matters what they eat. Let's give them the information they need to make good choices about food. Kids deserve better. Spinach deserves better.

"I'm strong to the finish cuz I eats me spinach! I'm Popeye the Sailor Man."

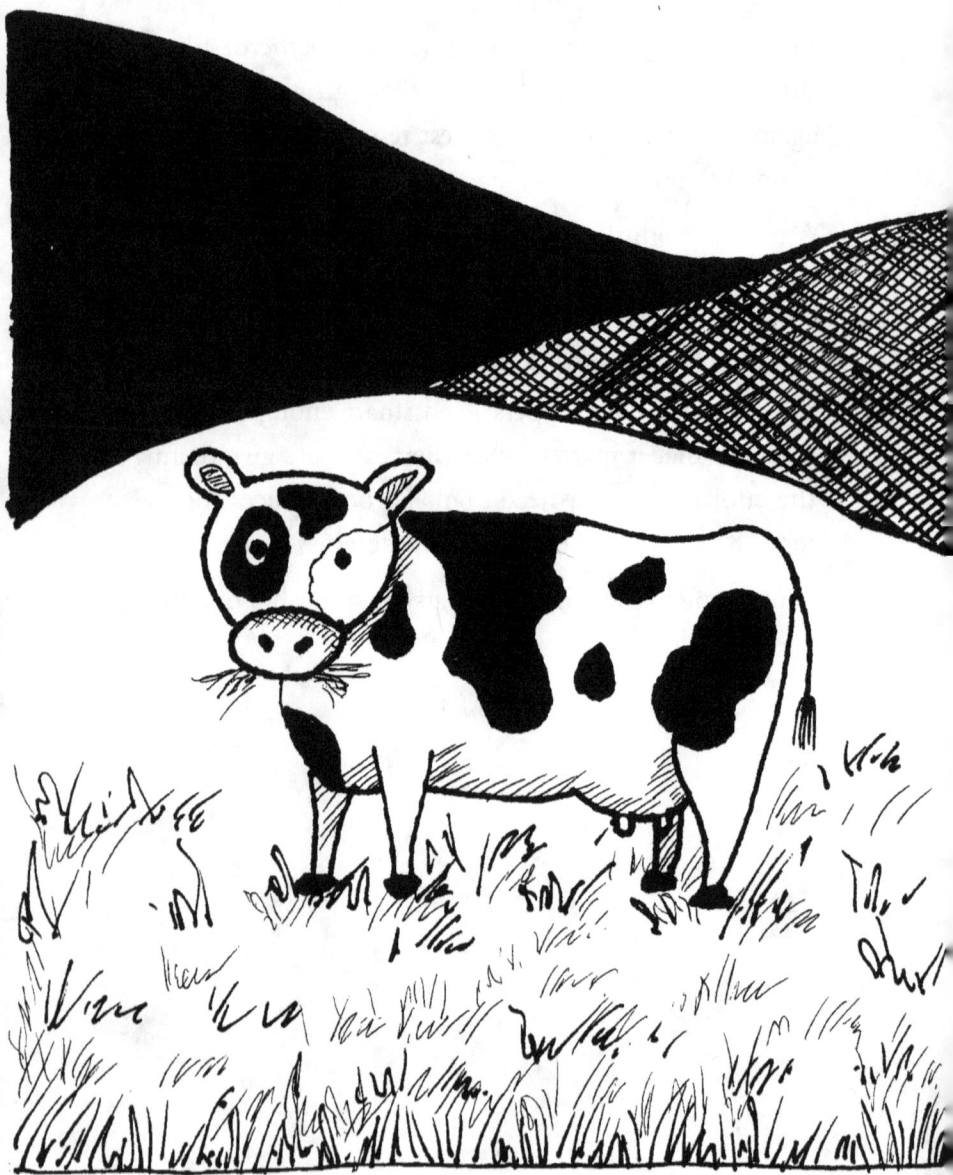

What to do in the Meantime

It could take a while to get your picky eater to the point where they really enjoy eating healthfully, so what can you do in the meantime? Here are a few ideas that will help you build up their immune system while you teach them a love of healthy foods.

Let Cows Eat Their Vegetables for Them!

Cows raised on factory farms are fed an unnatural diet of processed foods made mostly of corn and soy. This means the meat from these animals is missing the essential nutrients that your body needs. If your meat comes from cows raised naturally in a pasture, you get all the benefits of the hundreds of green leafy vegetables the cows graze on all day. Meat from a cow raised on a pasture may cost you more, but you're getting more. Those vitamins, minerals, and omega 3 fatty acids are worth every penny.

Let Chickens Eat Their Vegetables for Them!

You are what you eat eats. Read that again more slowly...you are what you eat eats. When you buy eggs from a factory farm the chickens are fed a diet of –you guessed it - corn and soy. Chickens are not vegetarians, they are omnivores, meaning they eat meat (worms, bugs etc...) and they love green leafy vegetables. If your chickens roam a pasture eating greens all day, you get the benefit of those veggies when you eat them! Caution: You want to look for eggs from pasture raised chickens, not "Pasteurized" which mean they've sterilized the egg, and not "Free Range" which used to mean the chickens were in a pasture until large corporations got their hands on the term. Now "Free Range" typically means there's a tiny door that leads to a dirt pen.

Hide Their Vegetables

There are lots of creative ways to add veggies to your child's diet that go unnoticed. Here are a few great tips...

Weekly Veggie Bin: Buy a couple bunches of kale, red leaf lettuce, spinach, or a combination of all three. Wash them and spin them dry in a salad spinner. Put them in a large container in the fridge. This makes it easy to add green leafy vegetables to sandwiches and salads. As little as ½ cup of green leafy vegetables per day can dramatically boost your immune system.

Hidden Recipes: Try the recipes in the next section. They are great tools for hiding veggies so kids will eat them.

Parsley Sprinkles: Keep fresh parsley on hand and when you're making a meal for your child sprinkle a little on top. Start with a very small amount and when they are comfortable with that keep adding a little more over time. Parsley is high in antioxidants, vitamins, minerals, and it helps remove toxins from the body.

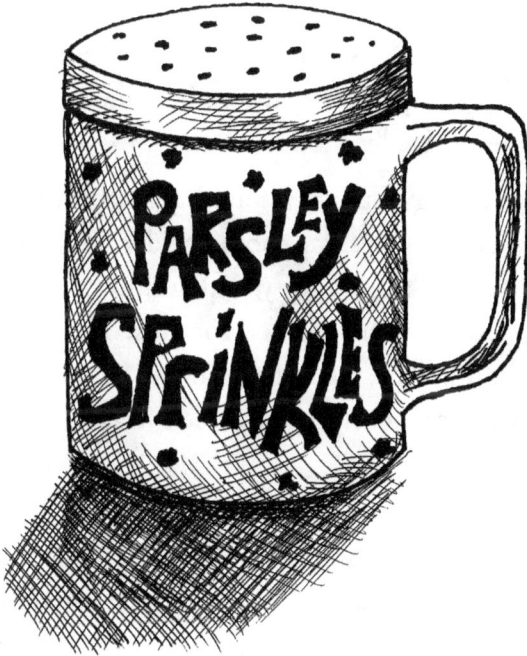

Kale or Spinach Sprinkles: You can add finely chopped spinach, kale or other greens to lots of foods and your kids won't even notice. Sprinkle them on frozen pizza and add them to canned soups, chili or spaghetti. Try putting micro greens or spinach on their sandwich instead of lettuce.

Micro Lettuce: You can buy pre-washed micro greens or baby spinach to add to their sandwich instead of lettuce.

Hidden in a Smoothie: Make a smoothie and throw in some spinach or kale. Not a lot. Just enough so it's in there but they won't notice.

Potato Pancakes: Most kids love potatoes, next time you make potato pancakes, throw in some freshly grated zucchini or finally chopped kale.

Avocado Pudding: This may sound crazy, but blend up a ripe avocado with some cocoa powder and maple syrup and you have a quick, easy, and healthy chocolate pudding. Avocados are so good for kids. They are loaded with healthy fats, vitamins, minerals, and antioxidants that are a real boost to your child's health.

We're Out of That, What About This?

Slowly work toward filling the house with lots of healthy options so your kids can eat anything they want…. but their choices are all healthy. As you are making the transition to healthier choices, it may be helpful to keep less junk food in the house. That way you naturally run out of items you're trying to cut back on at the end of the week. You're not depriving them of something they enjoy, but you're not making it a priority to always have it in the house either. "Michael we're out of Frosted Flakes, how about some home-made granola?"

Make Them Dessert

Another out of the box idea—one of the best ways to get your child to eat healthy is to make them dessert! The Internet is filled with desserts you can make with whole grains, fresh fruits...and yes, even vegetables. So don't be afraid to experiment—give the recipes in the next chapter a try. They're yummy.

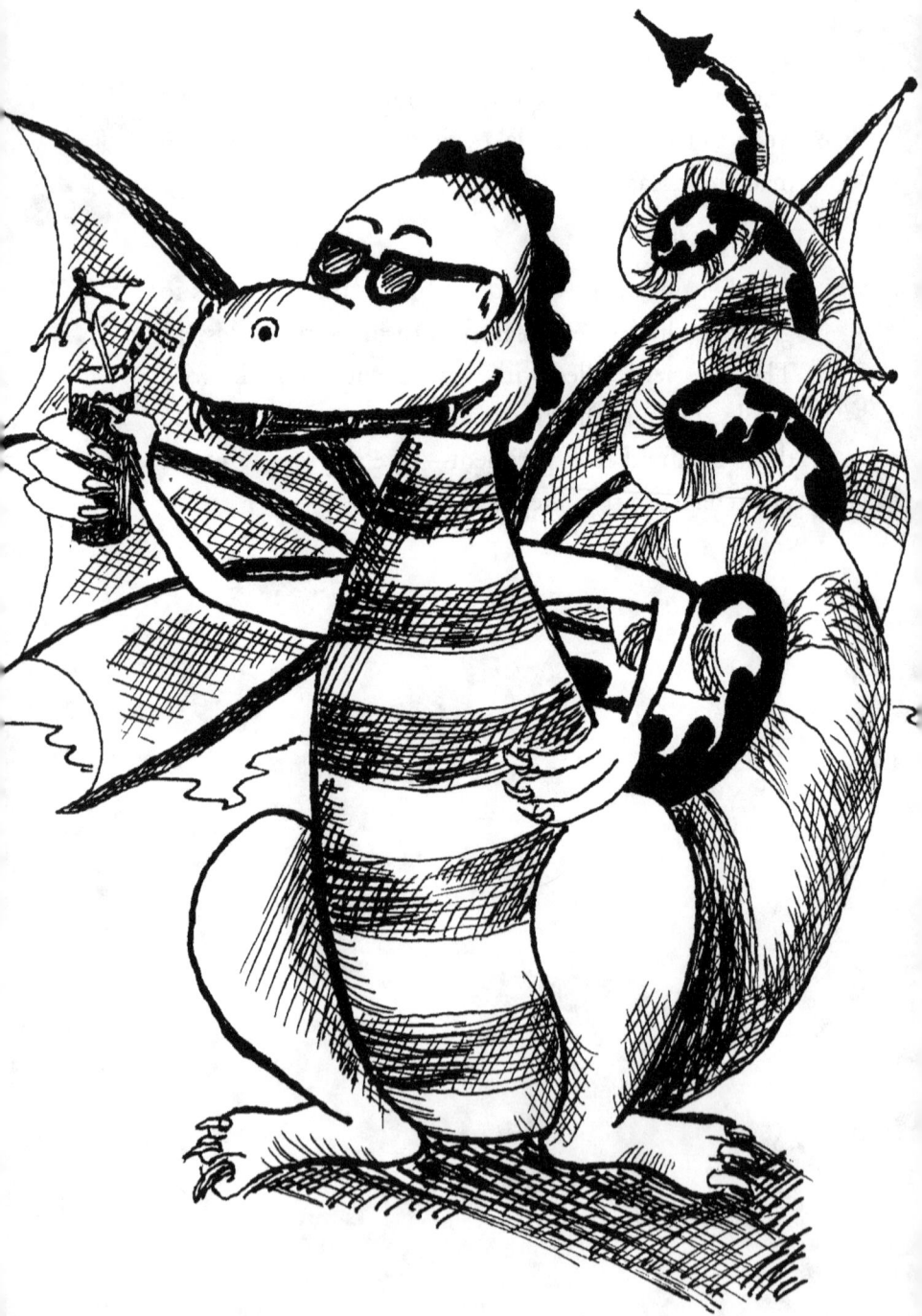

Crazy Veggie Recipes for Kids

Yes, these are crazy! Here's a few great recipes to launch your picky eater on an amazing food adventure.

Dragon Juice

Ingredients:

1 ripe sweet fresh pineapple well-chilled

2 leaves of green (not purple) kale

Tell your child you found a really crazy recipe for dragon juice. (If you have a really picky eater, invite a friend over that your child really admires and tell them their job is to get excited about making it and celebrate how wonderful the dragon juice is with you.) Juice the pineapple and the kale leaves in a vegetable juicer. Pour into fancy glasses and serve!

Zapple Pie

Instead of apple pie use chunks of zucchini in place of the apple! No one will know the difference.

Popeye Pesto

Use ½ Spinach and ½ basil the next time you make pesto. Let your kids help and when it's done let them spread it on crackers or dip pretzels into it.

Super Vegetable Stuffed Potatoes

Make twice-baked potatoes but throw finely chopped and sautéed broccoli or kale into the mix. Cover with cheddar cheese and bake.

Kale Chips

Let your child help make these. Wash kale and spin dry in a clean pillow case or salad spinner. Tear into little chips. Coat very lightly with salt and pepper or any other seasoning you like. Bake at 350 in the oven till crisp. Serve warm while everyone is watching a movie, or store in an airtight container to munch on throughout the week.

Rainbow Fries

I got this recipe from a friend when I was in graduate school in New England. They are fun to make and very yummy to eat!

1. Slice the following into French fry size pieces:

    1 Potato

    1 Turnip

    1 Sweet Potato

    1 Beet

2. Toss lightly with oil, chili power, salt and garlic powder.

3. Spread out across a large cookie sheet or baking pan and bake at 350 degrees for 30-40 minutes or until tender - stirring once half way through.

Eat as is or serve with a tasty dipping sauce of your choice. We love these plain or with a garlic aioli sauce for dipping!

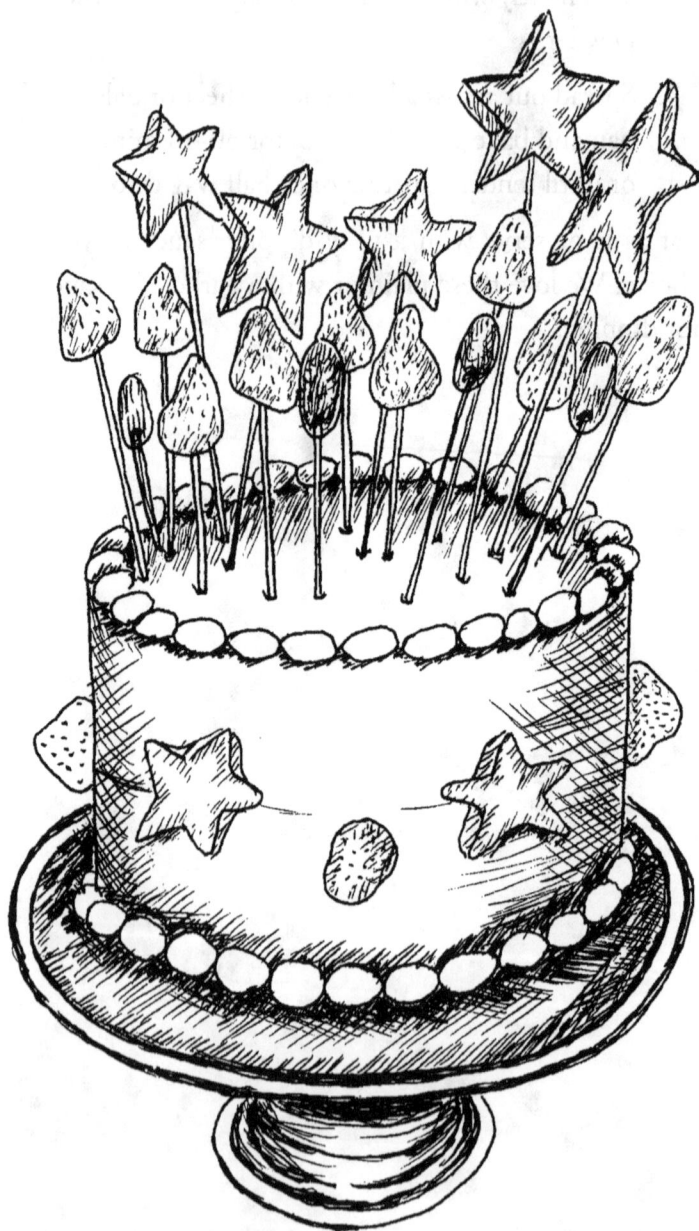

Healthy Desserts for Kids

What if you could give your child an amazing dessert that's actually really good for them? These dessert recipes are so healthy you could easily eat them for breakfast.

Watermelon Fireworks Cake

This cake is so much fun at a party, kids go crazy for it.

Ingredients:

1 large watermelon

1 star fruit sliced in thick slices that look like stars if available

Any assortment of the following for decorations:

Blueberries

Blackberries

Raspberries

Fresh, pitted bing cherries cut in half

Sliced apricot

Grapes

1. Make the cake rounds: Slice the watermelon into two big rounds the shape of a round layer of cake.

2. Remove the rind.

3. Stack the rounds to form a cake.

4. Decorate the top and sides with the fruit using toothpicks and wooden shish kebab skewers to attach them. If you use different sized skewers you can get the effect of a burst of fire works coming out of the top of the cake.

5. Enjoy!

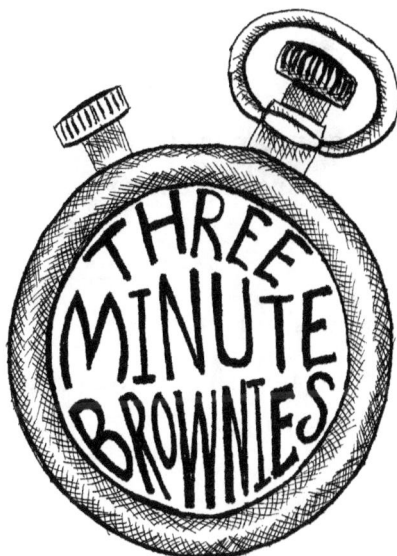

3-Minute Brownies

Ingredients:

8 pitted medjool dates

½ cup organic cocoa powder

½ cup raw organic almond butter

1. Blend the dates with the cocoa powder in a food processor until fine crumbs form. Don't over mix.

2. Add the almond butter and pulse until just combined. (For mint chocolate brownies, add some all natural mint flavor and pulse a few more times.)

3. Empty mixture into a bowl and form gently into little bite sized brownies. Don't compact the mixture, or it won't have that light baked feel to it.

OPTIONAL: Or, if you like, before you form the brownies, add any of the following flavorings: chopped walnuts, grated organic orange rind, fresh chopped rosemary, raw cocoa nibs, or anything else you like. Enjoy!

Incredible Crepes

This is one of my favorite recipes:

1   Cup fresh organic whole wheat pastry flour or whole organic oat flour

2   Eggs

1   Cup Milk

1   tsp. Salt

1. Beat all ingredients with a whisk until well combined.

2. Pour batter about 1/8th of a cup at a time into a small round skillet. Swirling the pan so that the batter THINLY coats the bottom.

3. You won't need to flip it. When it is golden brown on the bottom just peel it out of the pan and put it on a cutting board or plate to cool. I usually just bang the pan on my wooden cutting board and it flops out nicely. Repeat until all the batter is used up.

4. Fill with fresh or thawed frozen fruit mixed with real maple syrup to taste and top with freshly

whipped cream or vanilla yogurt. Very yummy! My kids will also just eat these plain as they come out of the pan. This recipe can be used for savory fillings at dinner as well.

A
Travel
Guide
for
Eating at Home

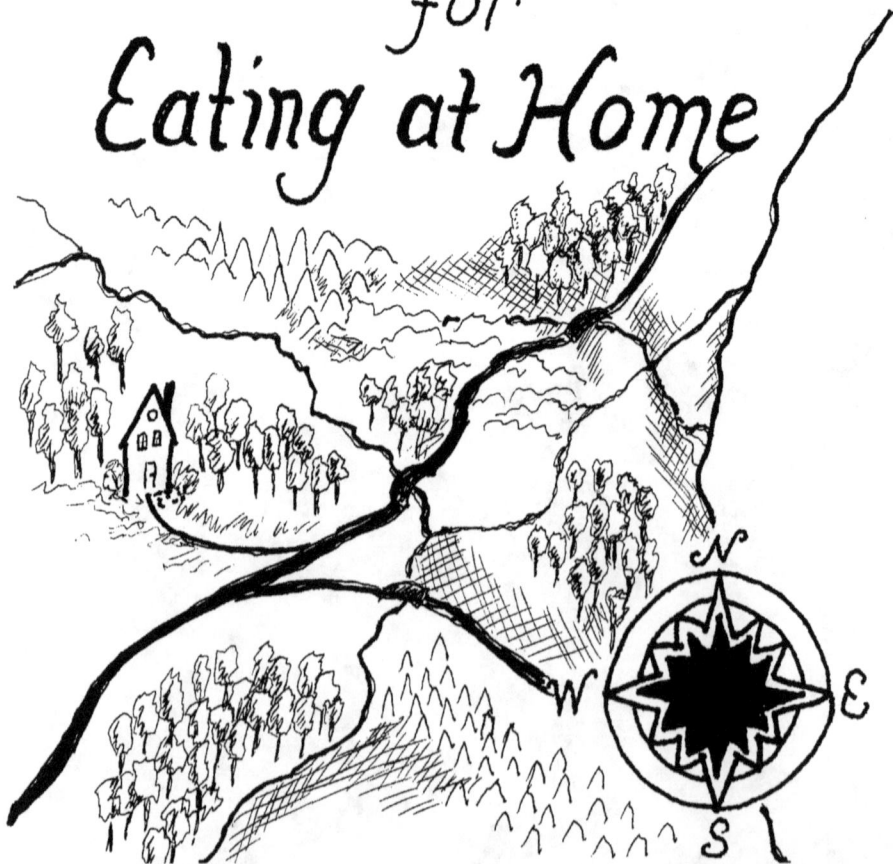

Eating at Home Made Easy

Here are some great tips to make eating at home easy for busy families:

Write it down

Sometimes there is amazing power in the simplest things. Knowing what you are going to make is half the battle when it comes to eating at home. Writing down what you're going to eat for the week on a meal planning sheet can be helpful in two ways:

First, it will help you know what ingredients you need when you go to the store.

Second, when you come home from work exhausted from your day you already know what you're going to make. In addition, knowing what you are going to make, means you can do a little prep work on the weekend or in the morning before you go to work.

Bring in the Troops

Don't try and do it all yourself. Get the kids involved making dinner in a meaningful way. Give them a way they can contribute their creative energy to the meal. (Remember what I said about that food chopper?) Make it easy for them the first couple of times with a new recipe by cutting up all the vegetables for them or getting out all the ingredients for them. This way, all they have to do is throw things in a bowl!

A great way to start is to get them to make the salad – even if they don't like salad. My kids would always say, "but I don't like that." My response… "You don't have to eat it if you don't care for it, you just have to make it because it's what we are having for dinner." Who knows, before long they might just pop a carrot or a slice of cucumber into their mouth as they're throwing it together.

If they are really little, prep the ingredients for them and let them decorate the salad with chopped veggies, nuts, olives, or cheese. They can become your "grand salad master." Then buy them their own salad cookbook!

Turn it Over Completely

When he's old enough, give your child the responsibility for making dinner for the family one night a week. I thought it would be more fun for my kids to choose what they wanted to make, and for some kids that might be true, but I found my boys disliked that part. So I choose a simple recipe that I know they'll like and I tuck the recipe and all the ingredients in a large container or bag in the fridge. Some of the ingredients I've

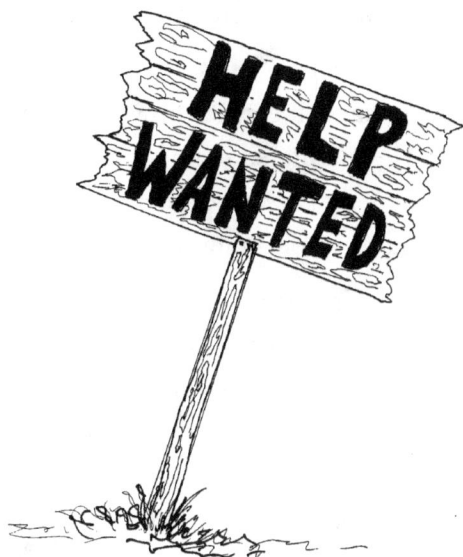

already prepped for them, like chopping the broccoli. All they have to do is pull out their bin and start cooking. I get to walk in the door to a home-cooked meal and they're gaining an incredibly valuable life skill.

Simple Sunday Prep

Sunday prep is a great life habit. You don't have to spend all day in the kitchen. You can spend anywhere from 10 minutes to 2 hours depending on your timeframe and still have a good head start for the week. Here are some examples of what you can do in a short amount of time.

10 Minute Sunday Prep: In just 10 minutes on Sunday you can wash a big bin of fresh vegetables, lettuce or salad greens, or marinate some chicken, beef or pork for the grill.

The salad bin makes it easy to throw a salad together all week long. The marinated meat can be quickly sautéed or grilled and makes a great dinner with some steamed broccoli or sliced whole grain bread.

1 Hour Sunday Prep: In one hour on Sunday you can make a big batch of meatballs and a bowl of curried chicken salad. If you double the meatball recipe you can freeze some for the following week. The chicken salad can be used for a topping on a green salad, for chicken salad sandwiches or as a snack on crackers. Use your bin of washed greens for the lettuce on the sandwich, as the foundation of the salad or to make curried chicken lettuce wraps for dinner.

2 Hours on Sunday Prep: With a little practice you can make enough food for the whole week in just two hours on a Sunday. Brown some ground beef, grate some cheese and layer up a lasagna. Cook up a batch of rice, sauté some vegetables and pork/chicken for a stir-fry or fried rice. Then layer some chicken, veggies and cheese between some corn tortillas for a nice Mexican casserole. With leftovers you'll have plenty for the whole week.

Week Day Morning Prep

Taking just a few minutes in the morning to make the salad or cook the rice is more helpful than you might think. Sometimes just having the meat browned for the taco or the rice made for the stir-fry is all you need to pull off a meal when you get home. It's so much easier to come home and cook if you have a partially made dinner waiting for you in your fridge.

Here are some other morning prep ideas...

Make the salad

Marinate the meat

Cook the pasta

Chop up the vegetables

Make the brown rice

Mix up the dry ingredients for biscuits

Make up the pizza dough, it can rise in the fridge all day

No Recipes

Instead of using recipes when you cook, just read cookbooks. Put a couple of cookbooks by your bed and flip through them at night. Nothing like a little food tour before going to sleep! Skim the ingredients list and you'll start to see patterns and the way different spices and ingredients go together. This will give you an intuitive sense of how recipes work. Then you won't need recipes to make dinner.

No Measuring

Stop measuring and start eyeballing your ingredients. It's easier, faster, and you have fewer measuring implements to clean up. Pour a teaspoon of salt into your hand. What does it look like sitting in your palm? Now do that instead of using a measuring spoon. A half cup of peanut butter is a pain to clean out, but it's about 3 big spoonful's so just ballpark it. Cooking becomes more of an art than a science, and a lot more fun.

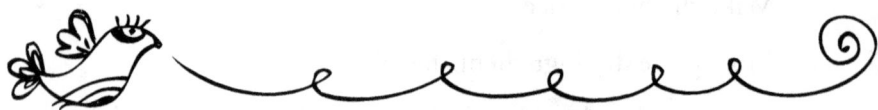

A Parent is one Who TEACHES A CHILD TO LOVE Healthy Food

The Purpose of Parenting

You are your child's support system and their teacher. You give them food, shelter, and a sense of belonging, but you also teach them how to survive and hopefully thrive in a complicated world.

When they're young, you're teaching them new things every day: the names of things, how to safely cross the street, what things they can and can't put in their mouths. Parents don't have any trouble teaching their children about things that are dangerous.

As a parent, it is important to understand the dangers of sugar in the body. As mentioned previously, consumption of sugar, not fat, is what drives inflammation in the body and what's known as metabolic syndrome. Metabolic syndrome is the precursor to a host of diseases including cancer, heart disease, type 2 diabetes, and dementia.

In addition to increasing inflammation, new research suggests that processed sugars also chemically block the hormones in your body like leptin that are responsible for telling your brain that you are full. This results in an urge to eat more, because your brain believes it's starving. When your body believes it's starving, it sends out signals that you should stop moving around to conserve energy—in short, eat more food, and don't get off the couch.

The processed food industry has put sugar into practically everything (80% of the foods lining the grocery shelves now have added sugar or corn syrup). If sugar is toxic to the body and an addictive substance, why are they putting it in all of our food? Two reasons: it's cheap and we crave it! It's cheap because as a society we heavily subsidize sugar and corn syrup, and we crave it because things in nature that are sweet, have in the past, always been good for us. Our bodies are not accustomed to sweet things that are toxic, so help your child realize the dangers of sugar, just like you do the dangers of crossing the street. It doesn't mean you can't cross the street, it just means you have to do so wisely. Teach your child not to eat sugar on an empty stomach. Reserve sweet treats for after a healthy meal with lots of natural fiber that will slow the absorption of the sugar into their system and help protect their liver.

NOTE: Right now, the processed food lobbyists are spending a lot of money to discredit the latest research on the effects of sugar and processed foods on the body. They're trying to confuse the public, but just like the tobacco companies, they won't be able to suppress the dangers much longer. For more on this research you can watch: **Fat Chance 2.0 with Doctor Robert Lustig here: http://bit.ly/FatChanceDrLustig**

3

House Rules

By Decree of the House of

(Your Family Name Here)

Thou shalt follow the herein written code of behavior. Any attempt to circumvent, change or disregard the stated rules below will be punishable by a dash through hot coals wearing a fake mustache and singing Lolita backwards!

1. No eating 1 hour before mealtime

2. thou shalt not say "yuck, Eww or Gross" at the dinner table!

3. All who reside within this dwelling shall at least taste not two, not three, but one tiny bite of each dish that some poor soul went to the trouble to prepare for you.

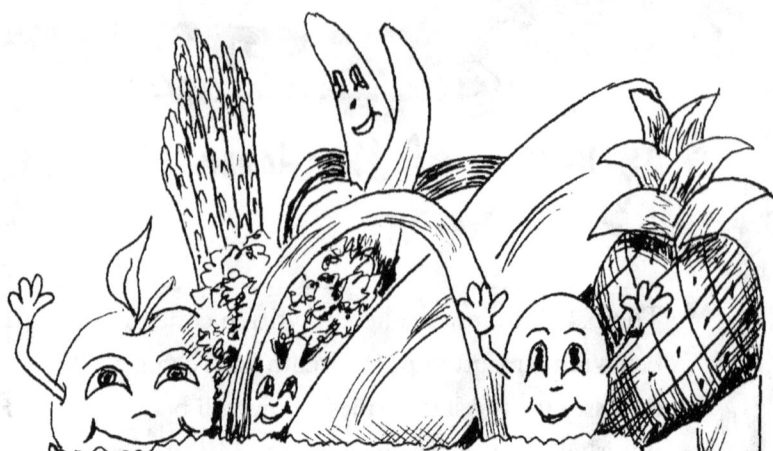

Shopping List

* Veggies
Fruits
Berries
Nuts
Seeds
Meat
Eggs
Whole Grains
Olive Oil
Yogurt
Whole Milk
Cheese

*Eat the most of these

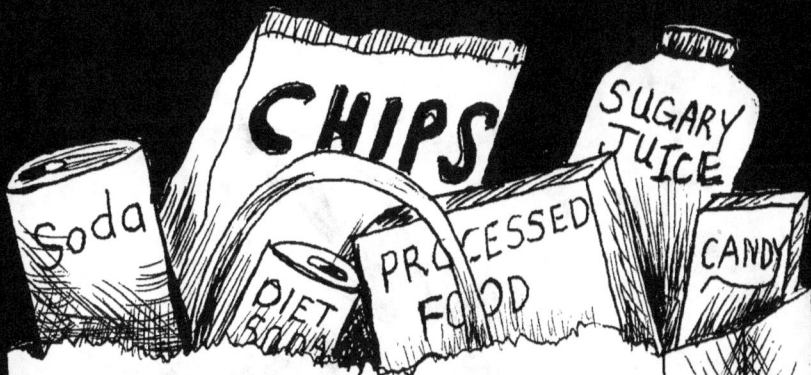

Anti-Shopping List

Soda

Diet Soda

Store Bought Juice

Fast Food

Processed Food

Kid's Meals

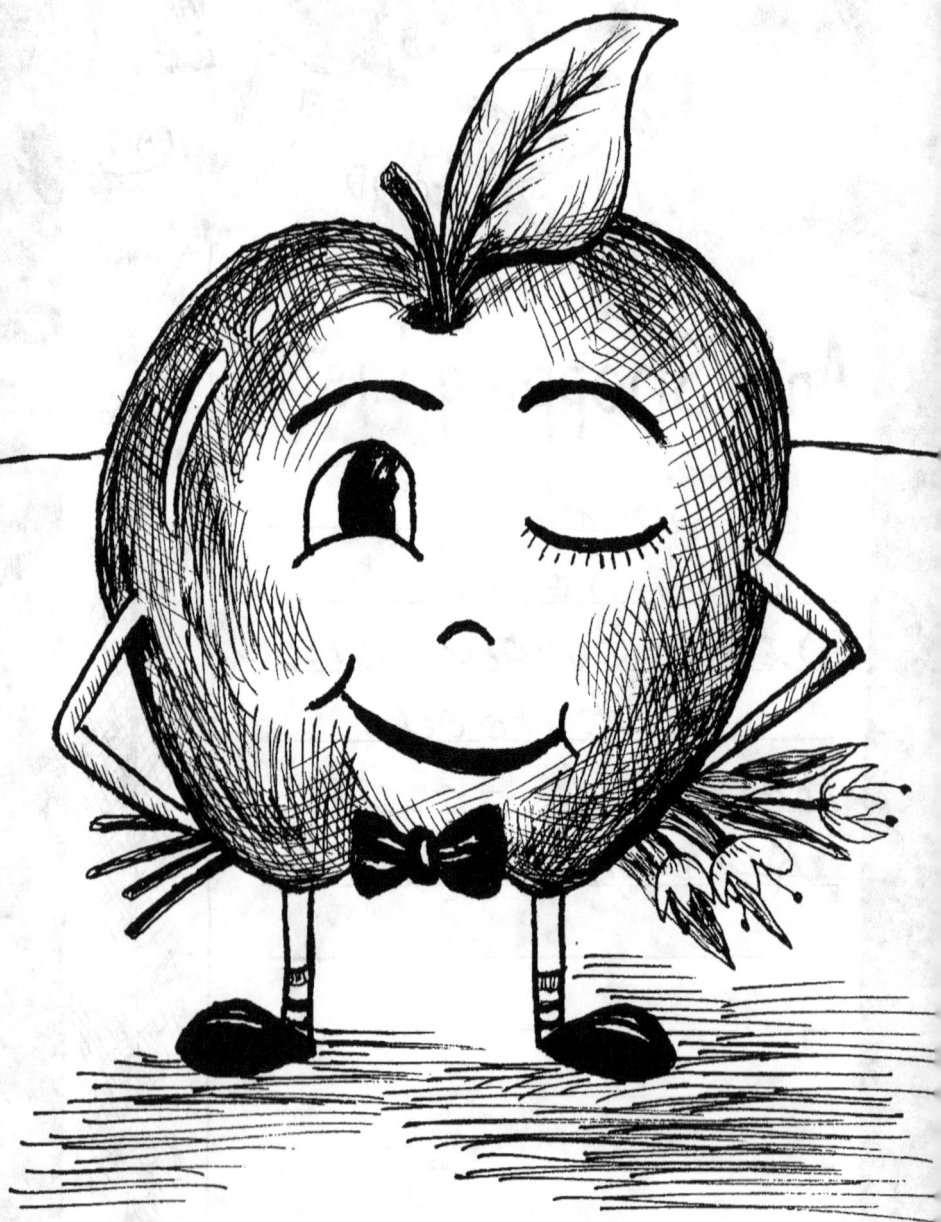

Sweets: To Eat or Not to Eat?

Bad For You, Avoid if you can:

Sugar

Brown Sugar

Fruit Juice Sweetened

High Fructose Corn Syrup

Corn Syrup

Artificial Sweeteners

Sweetened Beverages

Processed Fruit Juice

Better For You Than The Above, Small quantities:

Real Maple Syrup

Local Honey

Sucanat

Jaggery

Homemade Juice

Good For You, Eat as Much as You Want:

Fresh Fruit

Fresh Berries

Dried Fruit

NOTE: Spend some money here and get high quality in-season fruits that actually taste good. Fall grapes or spring strawberries are a great example. Head over to your local international store and give lychee or cherimoya a try. Take the kids apple picking in the fall or berry picking in the spring and summer. Order fresh citrus from a real orchard to cheer up the winter months!

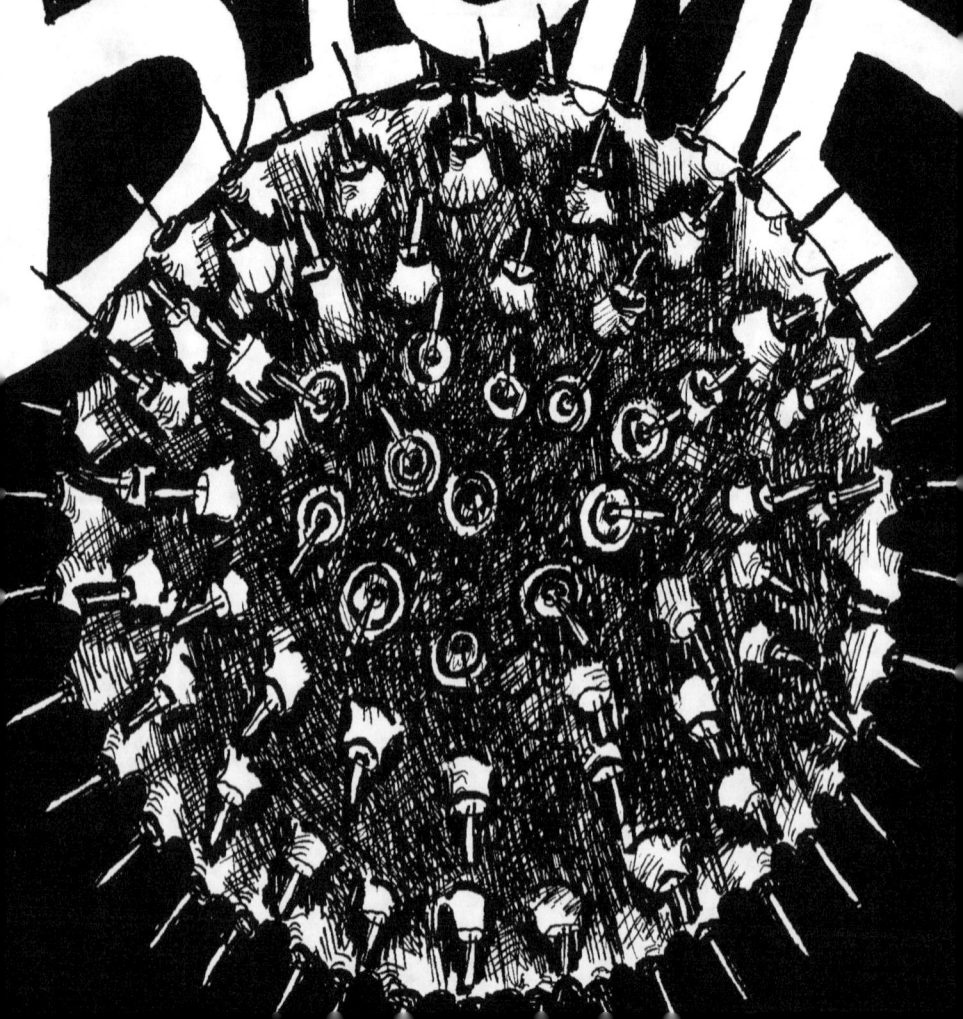

Meet Your Microbiome

Scientists and physicians are just now starting to understand the workings of your gut microbiome (colonies of micro organisms that live in your digestive tract).

These little guys are essential for your overall health. The types of microorganisms in your microbiome are determined by, among other things, what you eat. Eating processed foods builds a different type of microbiome in your gut than eating real food and some of these new organisms are not very good for you. In addition, new research suggests that your microbiome sends signals to your brain about what you crave to eat. If your child eats lots of processed foods, their microbiome will be sending them signals to eat more processed foods. These signals can be pretty strong, so it's up to us parents to support our kids in building a healthy microbiome, one that will help them crave healthy food.

Different ways you can build a healthy microbiome:

1. Eat whole foods, especially lots of vegetables.
2. Avoid antibiotics when possible.

3. Increase your consumption of natural fiber, eat more vegetables!

4. Eliminate or reduce your consumption of processed foods.

5. Eliminate or greatly reduce your consumption of sugar.

6. Take a high quality probiotic supplement.

7. Get outside, garden and let your kids play in the dirt!

8. Eat more garlic and leeks, which are great pre-biotics (food for your microbes).

9. Consume unprocessed, naturally fermented* foods like the following....

Pickles	Olives
Yogurt	Sauerkrut
Keefer	Kimchi
Naturally Fermented Breads	Beet Kavas

* *Make sure the label lists Naturally Fermented in the description.*

A healthy microbiome can help you…

- Digest your food
- Fight disease
- Produce serotonin
- Maintain a healthy body weight
- Nourish the cells that line your gut
- Avoid food allergies and asthma
- Protect your digestive tract

Often, feeding your child whole foods will build up their microbiome naturally, however in some cases more serious efforts are required as your child's gut lining may be damaged or there may be other issues that require attention first.

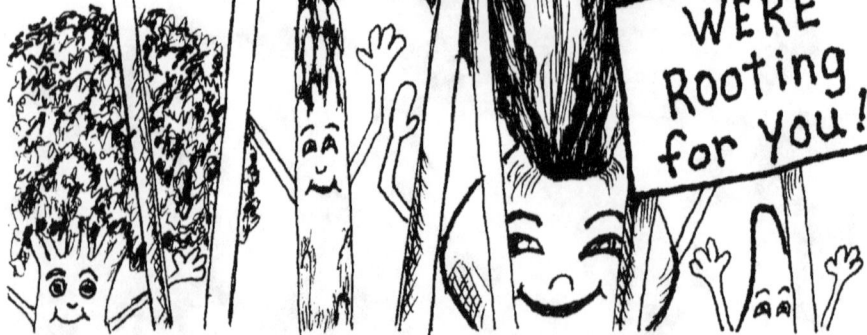

Quick Recap

Carry this around with you everywhere you go! Read it to yourself when you're brushing your teeth, recite it while you're driving in the car, and tattoo it just above your belly button.

Don't Give Up: You have 18 years to teach your child to eat healthfully, it's the greatest gift you can give them.

Back Sliding is Normal: It happens to everyone!!! Don't stress about it. Remember your kids will eat what they are used to. If you slide back into old habits, they will too! It will take some time to bring them around again. This even happens to adults, so give it some time to get back on track.

Preparing Ahead is Key: You'll only eat healthy if there is healthy around to eat, so prep ahead. Make 1 or 2 meals and a batch of healthy cookies on the weekend. Keep nuts and fresh fruit around and pack healthy snacks when you go on road trips.

Chicken Nuggets Are Not Food: Teach your children that candy, chicken nuggets, and processed mac & cheese are not food.

You Get To Decide: Remember, you are the parent and you get to decide what's for dinner, not your child. That's why your kids are not living in their own apartment. You have to teach them that it really does matter what they put in their bodies!

White Flour is Not Food: White flour and most processed foods have the majority of nutrients processed out of them. Put your energy into getting your child to eat nutrient rich whole foods like vegetables, berries, fruits, nuts, seeds, fish, meat, and real whole grains like oats and brown rice. It doesn't mean you can't eat white flour, just don't eat it thinking it's food and don't make it a staple of your diet.

Use Dairy in Moderation: Milk has growth hormones in it that are made to grow a 200 lb. calf to a 2,000 pound cow. Not such a good fit for a human. In addition, factory farmed cows are given added hormones to increase milk production, and lots of antibiotics to treat the infections the cows are getting from their poor diets and the strain on their immune systems. So use dairy products in moderation and buy products that are produced from cows that have grazed in a pasture.

Make Food Fun: Make sure family dinners are enjoyable. If this isn't happening on a regular basis, talk to someone and get it sorted out. Bounce your challenges off of a friend who's having some success. Talk to a counselor, or read through several of the parenting books in the reference section of this book. Your relationship with your child should not be unpleasant or confrontational. It should be enjoyable.

Take Care of Yourself: Your child will learn much more from what you do than what you say, so show your child how to take care of themselves. I've seen many lives changed forever by a serious illness. You don't appreciate how precious your health is until you or someone you love looses it. It's much easier to prevent an illness than to cure one, so put your health first, not soccer, not your job, not dance lessons. Slow your life down to the point that you have time to exercise and eat healthy. It will buy you a lot more time in the end. Research shows that a healthy diet and lifestyle can add as much as twelve good, productive years to your life.

Further Reading

Laurel's Kitchen
by Laurel Robertson

In Defense of Food
by Michael Pollan

Super Immunity for Kids
by Dr. Leo Galland

*How to Talk so Kids Will
Listen & Listen so Kids Will Talk*
By Adele Faber

Fat Chance
by Dr. Robert Lustig

The Discipline Book
by Dr. William Sears & Martha Sears, R.N.

Greene on Greens
by Bert Greene

References:

Many thanks to the wonderful authors listed below. I highly recommend each of these books to round out your healthy eating lifestyle and to help you raise happy, healthy, well adjusted kids!

Pollan, Michael. *In Defense of Food: An Eater's Manifesto.* London: Penguin, 2009.

Pollan, Michael. *Food Rules: An Eater's Manual.* New York: Penguin, 2009.

Chevat, Richie, and Michael Pollan. *The Omnivore's Dilemma: The Secrets behind What You Eat.* New York: Dial, 2009.

Edwards, Jaroldeen. *Things I Wish I'd Known Sooner: Personal Discoveries of a Mother of Twelve.* New York: Pocket Books, 1997.

Liedloff, Jean. *The Continuum Concept: In Search of Happiness Lost.* Massachusetts: Perseus Books, 1977.

Carper, Jean. *The Food Pharmacy: Dramatic Evidence That Food is Your Best Medicine.* New York: Bantam, 1988.

Willian, Sears MD. Martha, Sears R.N. *The Discipline Book: Everything You Need to Know to Have a Better-Behaved Child—From Birth to Age Ten*. New York: Little Brown and Company, 1995.

Lustig, Robert H. *Fat Chance: The Bitter Truth about Sugar*. London: Fourth Estate, 2013.

Moss, Michael. *Salt, Sugar, Fat: How the Food Giants Hooked Us*. New York: Random House, 2013.

Robertson, Laurel, Carol Flinders, and Brian Ruppenthal. *The New Laurel's Kitchen: A Handbook for Vegetarian Cookery & Nutrition*. Berkeley, CA: Ten Speed, 1986.

Faber, Adele, and Elaine Mazlish. *How to Talk so Kids Will Listen & Listen so Kids Will Talk*. New York: Scribner Classics, 2012.

Genetic and environmental influences on children's food neophobia1,2,3, The American Journal of Clinical Nutrition. August 2007vol. 86 no. 2 428-433

Can We Eat Our Way To A Healthier Microbiome? It's Complicated National Public Radio, November 08, 2013 4:17 PM ET by Maanvi Singh

Some of My Best Friends are Germs New York Times, May 15th 2013, by Michael Pollan

About the Authors

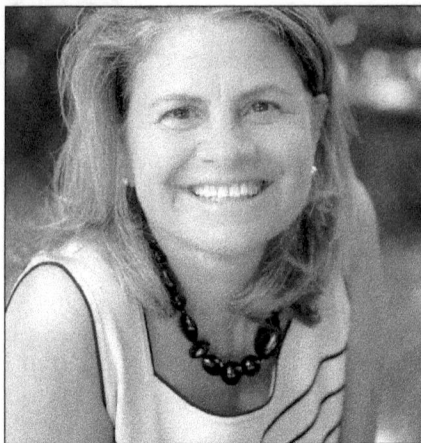

Beth Robeson 'the picky eater coach' has a Bachelor's Degree in Motivational Psychology and a Master's Degree in Sociology and has spent the last 25 years researching, writing and teaching families how to enjoy being healthy. She is an experienced public speaker and the creator of the "Picky Pirates 30-Day Program." While homeschooling two boys, Beth has been a stay at home and a working mom and understands the challenges of both. She has worked extensively with picky eaters, appreciates the power of a sweet tooth, and the importance of teaching kids to take responsibility for their own health. She speaks around the county and works directly with families to overcome the challenges of raising a child who is sensitive to the tastes, textures, and the look of food. To contact Beth about a speaking engagement or a consultation please e-mail her at beth@pickyeatercoach.com

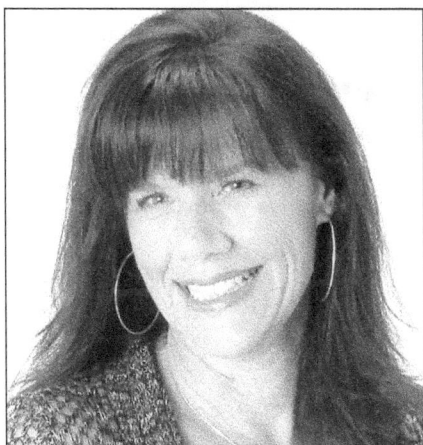

Charlene Ross is a freelance writer and blogger who looks for humor in all of life's situations. She lives in the suburbs of Los Angeles with her husband and two re-covering picky-eater teenage children. She will some-times smugly pat herself on the back when her seven-teen-year-old son requests salmon and grilled asparagus or her fourteen-year-old daughter takes a second serving of broccoli. And then she will remember the 5,482,687 chicken nuggets they consumed from toddlerhood well into their elementary school years and wipe that smug smile right off her face. She enjoys reading, listening to music, lingering over good food and wine with family and friends, and laughing. Always laughing. Check out her blog www.charleneaross.com

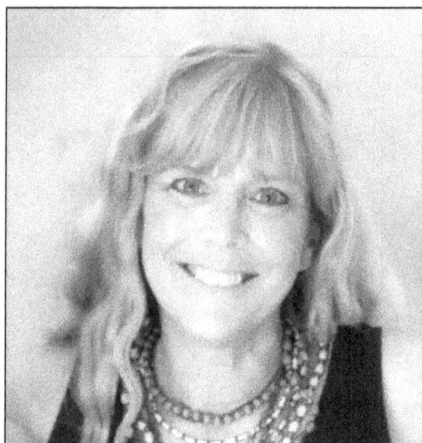

Lisa Boys is a prolific artist who's work spans many different types of media including drawing, painting, sculpture, and textiles. She is a graduate of the University of Cincinnati's Design, Art, Architecture and Planning program (DAAP) in fine arts. She specializes in custom works for clients, often using her talents to produce pieces that mark meaningful events in their lives. Lisa combines her passion for art with community service and teaching. For the past 15 years she has been teaching art classes for a wide range of students at the homeschool program Leaves of Learning and also teaches art at the Skyward Academy, a program for students with autism spectrum disorder. To contact Lisa about her work please e-mail her at lisamae2362@yahoo.com

Special Thanks

If you want to go fast go alone, if you want to go far, go together—African Proverb

Thanks to my boys, Kalen and Aaron who put up with endless requests to try a new recipe or one of my new "How-to-Get-Kids-To-Eat-Vegetables" techniques.

Thanks to my extended family and friends for helping edit and proofread this book, when I couldn't afford the cost of a traditional editor. On that note, special thanks to Madeline Shaw, Rachel Vaughn, Mikaela Vaughn and my Mom (what project would be complete without a little help from your Mom!)

Thanks to Todd Uterstaedt, a dear friend and mentor who gave me the courage to embrace my gift of writing.

Elise Donabedian, Nichole Foreman, thank you both for reading the first drafts of the book and giving me valuable insights as moms who are trying to raise healthy kids in this age of fast and tasty processed food.

Finally, thanks to my co-author Charlene Ross who helps bring on the funny as the words unfold, and my amazing illustrator Lisa Boys who brought the book to life with her beautiful and right-on-target sketches.

If you have a crazy picky eater parenting story to share, e-mail it to me at beth@pickyeatercoach.com and we may include it in our next book!

www.ingramcontent.com/pod-product-compliance
Lightning Source LLC
Chambersburg PA
CBHW052210270326
41931CB00011B/2288